Sexually Transmis
Infections in Clinical Practice

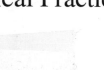

Alexander McMillan

Sexually Transmissible Infections in Clinical Practice

A Problem-Based Approach

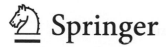 Springer

Alexander McMillan, MD, FRCP
Formerly, Consultant Physician
Department of Genitourinary
    Medicine
NHS Lothian,
Edinburgh Royal Infirmary, and
    part-time Senior Lecturer
University of Edinburgh
Edinburgh
UK
a.amcmm@btinternet.com

ISBN 978-1-84882-556-7   e-ISBN 978-1-84882-557-4
DOI 10.1007/978-1-84882-557-4
Springer London Dordrecht Heidelberg New York

British Library Cataloguing in Publication Data
A catalogue record for this book is available from the British Library

Library of Congress Control Number: 2009927018

Cover design: eStudio Calamar S.L.

Printed on acid-free paper

Springer is part of Springer Science+Business Media (www.springer.com)

Foreword

Patient care and training in the management of sexually transmitted infections has in recent years seen tremendous changes. A wider range of pathogens has been identified, tests streamlined with the introduction of newer technologies, evidence-based behavioural interventions introduced, and new therapeutic agents and vaccines developed. At the same time there has been a push to widen access to sexual health services and the development of protocol-based management where patients are often led through standardized histories and management guided by flow charts all performed by members of a mixed skilled and variously expert multidisciplinary team. Observing this process as an outsider either as a student or postgraduate trainee can be quite bewildering and much of the subtlety guiding management built into the processes can be lost unless one is working with expert clinicians who understand the theory and science underlying these strategies and are able to convey this to the trainee.

Book Title, *Sexually Transmissible Diseases in Clinical Practice*, provides a valuable resource to trainees in Sexual Health Medicine. It mimics the consultation process and although not an authoritative textbook on the subject provides the theoretical underpinning for management explained in an accessible way very much akin to sitting in on expert consultations in both common and some rarer conditions. It will also help trainees to prepare for Case Based Assessments (CBD) such as those required for training progression towards CCT in Genitourinary Medicine and guide preparation for the clinical OSCE component of the Diploma Examination in Genitourinary Medicine.

Raj Patel
2009

Preface

This book is aimed at several groups of health-care professionals who are involved in the care of individuals with or at risk of sexually transmissible infections.

With the relentless increase in the prevalence of the sexually transmissible infections in industrialized countries, and greater patients' expectations, most specialist clinics are under considerable pressure to provide a first-class service. One means of improving the performance of such clinics, particularly in the United Kingdom, has been to extend the role of the nurse practitioner. This has proved a most satisfactory solution in many clinics. It is hoped that this book will prove useful in the early training of the nurse practitioner through the presentation of a series of common clinical scenarios.

Problem-based learning has become the preferred teaching method in most universities, and it is hoped that undergraduate students will find the material presented here to be more than adequate to complement their clinical training in the management of sexually transmitted infections.

Postgraduate training in the specialty in the United Kingdom has undergone great changes over the past few years. By the end of the second year of specialist training, it is expected most trainees will have passed the examinations for the Diploma in Genitourinary Medicine, Society of Apothecaries, London. It is hoped that this book will give some assistance in the preparation for these examinations. In the United Kingdom, integration of Sexual Health services is the ultimate goal. Colleagues in disciplines related to Genitourinary Medicine, for example, Family Planning, should find the material presented a useful means of updating their knowledge of the sexually transmitted infections that they will be increasingly expected to manage. Clinical assistants who commence work in specialist clinics should also find the material presented here useful.

As access to specialist clinics may be difficult, many patients seek assistance from their general practitioner or practice nurse. It is hoped that this book will also prove useful to such health-care professionals.

The book is divided into two sections: Section A deals with the more common clinical scenarios that a competent practitioner should be able to manage, and Section B concerns more difficult cases and is more suited to those who have deeper knowledge about the infections. This book is not intended to be all-inclusive, but to focus on the practical aspects of patient care. A list of books and web sites from which detailed information on the epidemiology of the infections, the nature of the organisms involved, and their pathogenesis is found at the end of the book.

Alexander McMillan

Acknowledgments

I am grateful to my former colleague Dr Carolyn Thompson, Consultant Physician in Genitourinary Medicine, Edinburgh Royal Infirmary, for her advice on several case studies. Dr Kaveh Manavi, Consultant Physician in Genitourinary Medicine, Whittle Street Clinic, Birmingham, kindly provided Fig. 15.1. I am also grateful to Elsevier for permission to reproduce Figs. 2.1, 4.2, 5.1, 6.1, 7.3, 9.1, 9.4, 12.2, 18.1, 20.1, 23.1, 24.2, 25.1, 25.2, 30.1, 31.1, 31.2, 33.1 and 35.1 that appeared in *Clinical Practice in Sexually Transmissible Infections*, McMillan A, Young H, Ogilvie MM, Scott GR (eds.), 2002, Saunders, and Figs. 16.1 and 34.1 that were published in *Davidson's Clinical Cases*, Strachan MWJ, Sharma SK, Hunter JAA (eds.), 2008, Churchill Livingstone, pp. 73 and 80. Professor John Ackers, London School of Hygiene and Tropical Medicine, kindly permitted me to reproduce Figs. 10.1 and 31.1.

I am extremely grateful to Dr Imali Fernando, Consultant Physician, and Dr Sheena Lawson, Hospital Practitioner, Department of Genitourinary Medicine, Edinburgh Royal Infirmary, Edinburgh, UK who contributed Case Number 35.

I also wish to express my gratitude to the editorial staff of Springer-Verlag who provided invaluable support and encouragement.

Contents

Section B

Section A

Case 1
A Man Requesting a Sexual Health Screen

Robert, a 23-year-old student, attends a Sexual Health clinic and requests testing for sexually transmissible infections (STIs).

What History Would You Obtain from Robert?

A specific history should be taken to elicit any symptoms that the individual may not have recognized as being those of a sexually transmissible infection (STI) (It is usually helpful to elicit this history before enquiring about sexual activity: it helps to establish rapport with the patient before questioning about intimate activities). For example,

- Has he had discomfort on passing urine?

  o If so, consider urethritis.

- Has he noticed "growths" on the genitalia?

  o If so, consider genital warts, molluscum contagiosum, or normal anatomical variants, such as coronal papillae.

- Has he had an itch in the skin of the pubic area, genitocrural folds, shaft of the penis, scrotum, buttocks, or perianal region?

  o If so, consider phthiriasis and scabies, in addition to non-STI causes such as tinea cruris.

- Has he noticed swollen lymph glands in the groin (Fig. 1.1) or elsewhere in his body?

  o For example, painless inguinal lymph node enlargement may be a feature of primary syphilis and generalized

A. McMillan, *Sexually Transmissible Infections in Clinical Practice*,
DOI 10.1007/978-1-84882-557-4_1,
© Springer-Verlag London Limited 2009

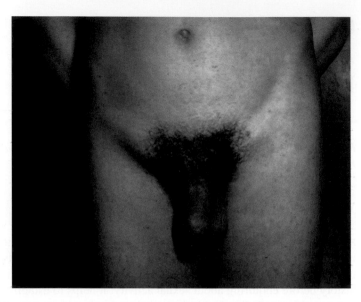

FIGURE 1.1. Bilateral inguinal lymph node enlargement in primary syphilis.

lymphadenopathy may be associated with secondary syphilis or HIV infection.

- Has he had testicular pain or discomfort? Some men with urethral chlamydial infection complain of testicular discomfort in the absence of frank epididymo-orchitis.

The taking of an accurate sexual history is important so that the most appropriate microbiological tests can be undertaken and the need for any subsequent investigations. The following information should be obtained:

- The date of his most recent sexual contact, and, if penetrative sex had been performed, were condoms used? (Remember the pre-patent periods of the STIs, e.g., gonococcal urethritis between 1 and 10 days and chlamydial urethritis 7–21 days. *Note*: Testing for STIs in the symptomless patient is generally deferred until 7–10 days after the most recent sexual risk.)

- Does he have a regular sexual partner, and, if so, for how long have they been in the relationship, and when did he last have sex with his partner? (Remember that one person's definition of "regular" may differ significantly from that of another!)
- If he has had sexual contact within the preceding 3 months:

  ○ How many different partners has he had?
  ○ What were the approximate dates of these sexual contacts? Again this is a relevant question with respect to the pre-patent periods of the infections.
  ○ What was the gender of these partners? Remember that a sizeable proportion of men who are predominantly hetero-sexual have had homosexual contact. If he has had homo-sexual contact, it is helpful to enquire about what sexual activities had occurred (see Case 4). This will inform on pos-sible risks of infection with, for example, HIV and syphilis.

- How many lifetime sexual partners has he had:

  ○ What was the gender of his partners?
  ○ Has he always used condoms for vaginal, anal, or oral–genital sex? Consistent use of condoms reduces the risk of infection with some, but not all, STIs. Examples of the for mer include gonorrhoea, chlamydia, and syphilis, and an example of the latter, human papillomavirus.
  ○ What was the country (countries) of origin of his sexual part-ner(s)? This is particularly important when considering the risk of infection with HIV, hepatitis B virus, and syphilis, conditions that are more prevalent in geographical areas out-with Western Europe, Australasia, and the United States of America.

- Has he had any STI in the past, and if so what, and when? This history is particularly important in the interpretation of positive serological tests for syphilis (see Cases 18, 19, and 33).
- Has he ever been tested for HIV, and if so when, and what was the result?
- Has he or any of his sexual partners ever injected recreational drugs? If so, it is important to note when that (these) risk(s) occurred because of the often long pre-patent period before serological tests for the blood-borne viruses become positive.

- Has he had any serious medical conditions in the past, and what is the current state of his general health?
- Is he currently receiving medication, and if so what? This is important to know because of possible drug interactions with any drugs used for the treatment of STIs.
- Has he taken any antimicrobial drugs within the preceding month? Such therapy may have inadvertently treated an STI.
- Has he ever had a hypersensitivity reaction to drugs, particularly to antimicrobial agents?

Robert has no symptoms suggestive of the presence of an STI. The reason for his clinic attendance is that he has met a young woman with whom he wishes to form a relationship, and does not wish to infect her with an STI of which he is unaware. His most recent sexual contact had been 3 weeks previously with an ex-girlfriend, with whom he had been in a relationship for 3 months. He used a condom for vaginal intercourse but not for oro-genital sex. He has had no other sexual contacts in the preceding 3 months. Each of his six lifetime sexual partners was female, and there is no history of homosexual contact. Each partner was from the United Kingdom. Although he is aware of the risk of acquisition of STI from unprotected sex, he has not used condoms consistently. He has smoked cannabis in the past, but has never injected recreational drugs. He is not aware of injecting drug use by any of his sexual partners. His general health is good, and he is not currently receiving any medication. There is no history of antimicrobial drug use in the preceding month. He has no known drug allergies. He has not been vaccinated against either hepatitis A or B.

Outline the Physical Examination You Would Perform and Indicate Which Microbiological Tests You Would Undertake in This Case

The extent of the physical examination will be determined by the history. As Robert has no history of a rash or swollen lymph nodes, it is reasonable to confine the physical examination to the anogenital area. This examination is best performed with the patient lying on a couch in a warm and well-lit room.

He should be offered a chaperone with whose gender he feels comfortable.

As up to 90% of men with uncomplicated chlamydial infection are symptomless, it is imperative that at least this infection is specifically looked for when a patient requests an STI screen. As gonococcal infection of the urethra is symptomless in up to 5% of cases, tests for *Neisseria gonorrhoeae* should be undertaken. Untreated, both infections have serious sequelae (see Cases 13 and 24).

1. Inspect the pubic area for, for example, *Phthirus pubis*, warts, and molluscum contagiosum.
2. Examine the genitocrural folds for tinea cruris or warts.
3. Palpate the inguinal lymph nodes. Non-tender inguinal lymph node enlargement may be a feature of primary syphilis (Fig. 1.1).
4. Palpate the testes and epididymes. Epididymo-orchitis may complicate untreated urethral chlamydial or gonococcal infections.
5. Examine the shaft of the penis. Identify lesions such as warts, molluscum contagiosum, and scabetic papules.
6. Retract the prepuce, if present, and look for warts or ulceration.
7. Examine the urethral meatus for urethral discharge. Evert the lips of the meatus to identify warts in the distal urethra.
8. In men with signs of urethritis (mucoid or mucopurulent urethral discharge with or without inflammation of the meatus), take material for Gram-smear microscopy as follows:

   a) Insert a plastic disposable inoculating loop (10 μL) into the urethra to a distance of about 3 cm, gently scrape the walls of the urethra, and withdraw the loop.
   b) Prepare a smear on a microscope slide.
   c) Stain the smear by Gram's method and examine microscopically (see Cases 5 and 7).

9. Urethral gonorrhoea is diagnosed or excluded as follows, depending on local clinic and laboratory practices:

   ○ Obtain material for culture for *N. gonorrhoeae* by gently inserting a disposable plastic inoculating loop (10 μL) into the distal 3 cm of the urethra, withdrawing, and inoculating a plate of selective culture medium, or

○ Obtain material using a cotton wool-tipped applicator stick and send to the laboratory in appropriate transport medium for culture, or

○ Send a first-voided specimen of urine to the laboratory for testing for *N. gonorrhoeae* by a nucleic acid amplification test. [1] (Combined assays for the dual detection of infection with *N. gonorrhoeae* and *C. trachomatis* are now available, and some laboratories can test for both infections on one urine sample), or

○ If the man is unable to provide a urine sample, urethral material for testing for *N. gonorrhoeae* by NAATs can be obtained by passing a swab, provided by the manufacturer of the test collection kit, about 3–5 cm into the urethra, withdrawing, and breaking off the end into a buffer solution. The dual detection NAATs are particularly helpful under these circumstances, as the need for two swabs is obviated.

○ (Some clinicians prepare a Gram-stained smear of urethral material collected as above for microscopy. The sensitivity of direct microscopy is low in symptomless individuals and in populations where the prevalence of gonorrhoea is low, such as in Robert's case).

10. Test for chlamydial infection, if not already done (see comments above on detection of gonococcal infection):

○ Send an aliquot (about 20 mL) of first-voided urine for the detection of *Chlamydia trachomatis* DNA by a NAAT.

○ If he is unable to provide a urine sample, urethral material for testing by a NAAT can be obtained as described above for gonorrhoea.

11. Offer serological testing for

○ Syphilis (for example, an enzyme immunoassay).

○ HIV infection.

---

[1] A positive result in a nucleic acid amplification assay should preferably be confirmed by culture or an alternative NAAT.

*Physical examination has failed to identify features of any STI;
a urine sample is sent for the detection of* N. gonorrhoeae *and*
C. trachomatis. *Robert accepts the offer of serological tests for
syphilis and HIV. He is asked to contact the clinic for the results of
the laboratory tests 1 week later.*

*At this time he contacts a Health Adviser. He is told that the test
results are negative and that there was no evidence on infection.
Robert, however, is uncertain as to the accuracy of the tests. What
information would you provide?*

Robert is assured that the tests for gonorrhoea and chlamydial infection are reliable. The sensitivity of NAATs is supe-
rior to culture for the diagnosis of urethral gonorrhoea in men.
Although the sensitivity and specificity[2] of polymerase chain reactions (PCRs) for *N. gonorrhoeae* are reported to be about 90 and
99.5%, respectively, for urine samples, the sensitivity is somewhat
lower in symptomless than in symptomatic men. Slightly higher
sensitivity (about 96%) is reported when urethral swabs are used
as specimens.

The sensitivity and specificity of PCRs for *C. trachomatis* are
about 84 and 99%, respectively, for urine samples. The sensitivity
compares well with that of about 88% for urethral swabs.

As the sensitivity, specificity, positive-predictive, and negative-
predictive values of NAATs for the diagnosis of infection using a
first-voided specimen of urine are similar to those using directly
obtained urethral material and does not involve invasive sampling,
this specimen is preferred for screening.

As his most recent sexual contact had been only 3 weeks before
testing, and the pre-patent period of syphilis varies between 10 and
90 days, Robert should be offered repeat testing in about 8 weeks
time if he is concerned. In this case the risk of syphilis is low
(most cases of syphilis in the United Kingdom have been acquired
through homosexual contact or from individuals who have traveled

---

2

True Positive	False Positive
w	x
False negative	True negative
y	z

Sensitivity = $w/(w + y)$. Specify = $z/(x + z)$
Positive predictive value = $w/(w + x)$. Negative predictive value = $z/(y + z)$

from geographical areas where the infection is prevalent), and it is probably unnecessary to insist on repeat testing.

As HIV antibodies may take up to 3 months from infection to become detectable, a negative test at this time cannot exclude infection. Robert should be offered re-testing in about 8 weeks time, although, as in the case of syphilis, the risk of HIV infection is low (most cases of HIV infection in the United Kingdom have been acquired through homosexual contact, from unprotected vaginal or anal sex with a person from a geographical area where HIV is prevalent, or from sharing contaminated equipment used for injecting recreational drugs).

Robert has read about inapparent genital herpes and asks why he has not been tested for this viral infection. He has never been aware of any genital or oral lesions suggestive of genital or oral herpes, and none of his sexual partners is known to have genital herpes. What would you tell Robert?

Robert is correct in his understanding that many cases of genital herpes are symptomless. Only between 10 and 25% of individuals with serological evidence of herpes simplex virus (HSV) type 2 infection are aware that they have genital herpes (worldwide, HSV type 2 is the most common type associated with genital infection). In the absence of clinical lesions that can be sampled for virological testing (see Case 16), serology remains the only means for detecting infection. Type-specific glycoprotein G (gG)-based assays are available that have sensitivities for the detection of HSV-2 antibodies of between 80 and 98% and specificities greater than 96%. The positive-predictive value (see Note 2), however, is poor in low prevalence populations. There is a good correlation between the seroprevalence of HSV type 2 and increasing age, the number of years of sexual activity, and the number of sexual partners. As Robert is young, has been sexually active for a short period of time, and has had few sexual partners, a positive result from his serum does not necessarily reflect true infection.

In some industrialized countries, including the United Kingdom, almost 50 and 70% of new genital herpes infections are associated with HSV type 1, the viral type classically associated with orolabial herpes. As in the case of genital infection with HSV type 2, more than one-third of orolabial infections are symptomless. In the absence of a history of oral or genital lesions it is therefore impossible to tell whether the detection of HSV type 1 antibodies reflects orolabial or genital herpes.

Opinion is divided as to whether or not HSV type-specific serology should be part of a sexual health screen. On the one hand, infection is lifelong, there is no curative treatment, and the psychological morbidity associated with a diagnosis of HSV type 2 infection can be profound. On the other hand, however, seropositive individuals can be taught to recognize minor recurrences and avoid intercourse at that time, thereby reducing, but not eliminating, the risk of transmission to a partner. With adequate support, the psychological impact is usually short lived. Persons with HSV type 1 antibodies should be advised to avoid oral–genital sex with a partner who has no history of orolabial herpes, or who is not known to be seropositive for that viral infection.

After this discussion, Robert does not wish to be tested for type-specific HSV antibodies.

Case 2
A Woman Requesting a Sexual Health Screen

Mary, a 28-year-old dental receptionist, attends a Sexual Health clinic requesting testing for sexually transmissible infections (STIs). She has just discovered that her ex-partner had had other sexual contacts during the time they were in the relationship.

What History Would You Obtain from Mary?

A specific history should be taken to elicit any symptoms that the individual may not have recognized. For example,

- Has she noticed increased vaginal discharge?

    ○ This may be physiological or associated with an STI such as *Trichomonas vaginalis*.

- Has she noticed "growths" on the genitalia?

    ○ If so, consider genital warts, molluscum contagiosum, or normal anatomical variants, such as pilosebaceous glands.

- Does she have itch in the skin of the pubic area, genitocrural folds, labia majora, introitus, perineum, buttocks, or perianal region?

    ○ If so, consider phthiriasis, scabies, candidiasis, or a non-STI such as a genital dermatosis (Fig. 2.1).

- Has she noticed post-coital bleeding or inter-menstrual bleeding?

    ○ If so, consider chlamydial infection.

A. McMillan, *Sexually Transmissible Infections in Clinical Practice*,   13
DOI 10.1007/978-1-84882-557-4_2,
© Springer-Verlag London Limited 2009

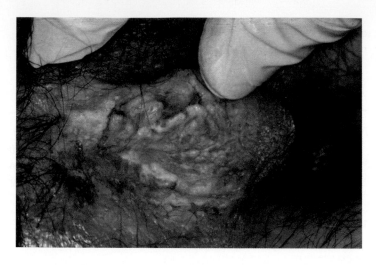

FIGURE 2.1 Lichen simplex of labium minus

- Has she had lower abdominal pain and/or deep dyspareunia?

  ○ These may be features of pelvic inflammatory disease (PID) that may be caused by chlamydial or gonococcal infections. Irregular menstrual bleeding may be an additional feature of PID.

- Has she had frequency of micturition with or without dysuria?

  ○ Chlamydial and gonococcal infections can be associated with these symptoms, as may a urinary tract infection.

- Has she noticed swollen lymph glands in the groin or elsewhere in her body?

  ○ Painless inguinal lymph node enlargement may be a feature of primary syphilis, and generalized lymphadenopathy may be associated with secondary syphilis or HIV infection.

The details in the sexual history do not differ significantly from those described in Case 1 for the heterosexual man. Early in the consultation it should be established if her partners are male or female. Note should be made of the date of her last menstrual period, and the menstrual cycle should be recorded. The method of contraception used, if any, and an obstetric history should be noted. It is also helpful to know the date of her most recent cervical smear and the result.

Mary has no symptoms suggestive of the presence of an STI. Her most recent menstrual period had been 2 years previously – she had been fitted with a progestogen-only implant (Implanon®) for contraception. Her most recent sexual contact had been 4 months previously with her ex-partner with whom she had been for 3 years. As she thought that her partner was faithful, condoms were not used during sexual intercourse. She has had no other sexual partners during that time, and she has had only one other lifetime partner with whom she had separated 6 years previously. Both partners were British, neither they nor she has injected recreational drugs, and neither man is known to have had homosexual contact. She has had no female sexual partners. Her general health is good, and she is not currently receiving any medication other than Implanon®, and she has not been treated with antimicrobial drugs within the preceding month. Since the age of 20 years, Mary has had 3-yearly cervical cytology examinations, the most recent having been 6 months previously, and no abnormalities have ever been reported. She has had one pregnancy that was terminated 3 years previously.

Outline the Physical Examination You Would Perform and Indicate Which Microbiological Tests You Would Undertake in This Case

The extent of the physical examination will be determined by the history (see Case 1). As Mary has no history of a rash or swollen lymph nodes, it is reasonable to confine the physical examination to the anogenital area. The examination should be performed with the woman in the semi-lithotomy position on a couch in a warm and well-lit room. A presence of a chaperone should be offered and one must be present when a male doctor undertakes the examination.

As the majority of women with uncomplicated gonococcal and chlamydial infections are symptomless, it is imperative that at least these infections are specifically looked for when a patient request an STI screen. Untreated, both infections have serious sequelae (see Cases 14, 24, 27).

1. Inspect the abdomen, and palpate for tenderness, guarding, and masses; note should be made of enlargement of the liver or spleen.
2. Inspect the pubic area for, for example, *Phthirus pubis*, warts, and molluscum contagiosum.
3. Palpate the inguinal lymph nodes, and note enlargement such as may occur in primary syphilis.
4. Inspect the labia majora for lesions such as warts or ulcers, or for a genital dermatosis (Fig. 2.1).
5. Gently separate the labia minora from the labia majora. Examine the labia minora and, after wiping with a cotton wool ball, inspect the introitus. Look particularly for warts and lesions of herpes simplex virus.
6. Urethral gonorrhoea is diagnosed or excluded as follows, depending on local clinic and laboratory practices:

   ○ Obtain material for culture for *N. gonorrhoeae* by gently inserting a disposable plastic inoculating loop (10 μL) into the distal 1 cm of the urethra, withdrawing, and inoculating a plate of selective culture medium. Or,
   ○ Obtain material using a cotton wool-tipped applicator stick and send to the laboratory in appropriate transport medium for culture. Or,
   ○ If a nucleic acid amplification test (NAAT) [1] is used for the detection of *N. gonorrhoeae*, obtain urethral material using the swab provided by the manufacturers of the test kit, break it into the buffer solution, and send it to the laboratory. (This test may be omitted if a NAAT is used for testing cervical material)
   ○ Some clinicians prepare a Gram-stained smear of urethral material collected as above for microscopy. The sensitivity

---

[1] A positive result in a nucleic acid amplification assay should be confirmed by culture.

of direct microscopy is low in populations where the prevalence of gonorrhoea is low, such as in Mary's case.

Note: In many clinics serving populations with a low prevalence of gonorrhoea, testing for urethral infection has been abandoned.

7. Pass a plastic bivalve vaginal speculum and examine the character of any vaginal discharge. For example, typically in bacterial vaginosis, there is a homogeneous milky-white discharge that coats the vaginal walls. Note inflammation of the vaginal walls, as may occur in trichomoniasis.
8. Collect a sample of material using a 10 μL plastic inoculating loop from the posterior vaginal fornix (or lateral fornices if candidiasis is suspected).

   ○ Prepare a smear on a microscope slide for subsequent Gram staining, and then suspend some of the material in a drop of isotonic saline on another slide.
   ○ Examine (oil immersion lens, magnification ×1,000) the Gram-stained smear, noting the presence or absence of lactobacilli (see Case 9).
   ○ Examine (magnification ×400) the saline-mount preparation for the motile trophozoites of *T. vaginalis*, fungal hyphae or "pseudohyphae," and "clue cells" (see Cases 9, 10, 25 and 26).

Note: Facilities are available in some clinics for the detection of trichomonal infection by culture or NAAT. Vaginal specimens should be processed according to the instructions from the local laboratory.

9. Note the appearance of the ectocervix and the character of any discharge from the endocervical canal; in chlamydial and gonococcal infections, for example, there *may* be a mucopurulent discharge.

   ○ In the majority of women with chlamydial infection the cervix appears normal.

- ○ The cervix may appear normal in women with gonococcal infection, but sometimes a mucopurulent discharge may be observed.

10. Cervical gonococcal is diagnosed or excluded as follows, depending on local clinic and laboratory practices:

- ○ Obtain material for culture for *N. gonorrhoeae* by gently inserting a disposable plastic inoculating loop (10 μL) into the distal 1 cm of the endocervical canal, withdrawing, and inoculating a plate of selective culture medium. Or,
- ○ Obtain material using a cotton wool-tipped applicator stick and send to the laboratory in appropriate transport medium for culture. Or,
- ○ If a nucleic acid amplification test (NAAT) (see Note 1) is used for the detection of *N. gonorrhoeae*, obtain endocervical material using the swab provided by the manufacturers of the test kit, break it into the buffer solution, and send it to the laboratory.
- ○ Some clinicians prepare a Gram-stained smear of endocervical material collected as above for microscopy. Although the sensitivity is low in low prevalence populations, microscopy may be useful if mucopus exudes from the endocervical canal. If Gram-negative diplococci are seen, a *presumptive* diagnosis of gonorrhoea can be made and treatment given without delay.

11. Collect endocervical material for the detection of *Chlamydia trachomatis*-specific DNA sequences (by a NAAT), using the swab provided by the manufacturers of the test collection kit. The swab is inserted into the endocervical canal to a distance of about 1 cm. After rotating the swab once in the canal, it is withdrawn and the end broken off into the buffer solution provided.

Note: Some laboratories now use a single test for the dual detection of *N. gonorrhoeae* and *C. trachomatis*, obviating the need for two swabs.

12. Inspect the perineum, perianal region, and anus for lesions such as warts.
13. If there are symptoms of proctitis, specimens for the diagnosis or exclusion of gonorrhoea and/or chlamydial infections are collected as described in Case 3.
14. Offer serological tests for

   ○ Syphilis;
   ○ HIV infection.

Mary has no clinical abnormalities suggestive of an STI. Microscopy of a saline-mount preparation of vaginal material does not show T. vaginalis. *In the Gram-stained smear from the vagina, lactobacilli are the predominant flora, and only a few polymor phonuclear leucocytes are seen. Microscopy of urethral and cervical material is not undertaken. Cervical material is sent to the laboratory for testing for both* N. gonorrhoeae *and* C. trachomatis *by a NAAT. She accepts serological tests for syphilis and HIV infection. She is advised to telephone for the test results in 1 weeks' time.*

At that time, she telephones a Health Adviser in the clinic to discuss the results. Although all the tests are negative, she wants to find out about the reliability of these "new tests" for gonococcal and chlamydial infections. She also asks why a cervical specimen was obtained, as a friend from overseas had only provided a urine test for these infections. How do you respond?

Nuclei acid amplification assays, including polymerase chain reactions (PCRs), have been shown to be more sensitive than culture for the diagnosis of gonorrhoea in women. The sensitivity of PCR for cervical specimens is between 92 and 99%, compared with about 60% for culture; the specificity of the PCRs is almost 100%. In the diagnosis of chlamydial infection by NAATs on cervical material, the sensitivity is about 86% and the specificity is almost 100%.

With respect to urine testing for chlamydiae, the sensitivity (83%) is only slightly less than for cervical specimens, making this a convenient sample for screening. The sensitivity of NAATs on urine samples for the detection of gonococcal infection, however, is significantly lower (about 56%) than on cervical material. Urine testing for gonorrhoea therefore cannot be recommended.

Case 3
A Female Sex Industry Worker Requesting a Sexual Health Screen

Two years later, Mary re-attends the clinic. She tells you that for the past 3 months she has been providing "escort services," including sex. Although she is symptomless she requests testing for STIs. Her most recent sexual contact with a client had been about 10 days previously, and she had provided protected oral–genital and vaginal intercourse. Over the preceding 2 months she has had sexual contact with about five different clients per week, some men having been from South-East Asia. Clients use condoms consistently for vaginal sex but condoms are not always used for oral–genital sex. She has also been in a regular relationship for 18 months with a male partner who does not use condoms for intercourse. She does not use recreational drugs, but she does not know if any of her clients have ever injected such drugs. The Implanon® had been replaced about 1 year previously. Her general health remains good and she is not receiving any other medication. She has had no further pregnancies.

What Tests Would You Undertake Now, and Against Which Infection Might You Consider Vaccinating Her?

The tests that were performed at her initial clinic attendance should be undertaken. In addition:

A. McMillan, *Sexually Transmissible Infections in Clinical Practice*,
DOI 10.1007/978-1-84882-557-4_3,
© Springer-Verlag London Limited 2009

- Take a pharyngeal specimen for culture or examination by a NAAT[1] for *N. gonorrhoeae*. A cotton wool-tipped applicator stick is passed over the pharynx and both tonsils or tonsillar beds, and either plated directly on to selective culture medium or sent to the laboratory in the appropriate transport medium. The majority of individuals with pharyngeal infection are symptomless, but, untreated, there is the possibility of transmission to a sexual partner, and the woman is at risk for disseminated infection (see Case 24). Some studies have shown that, among female sex industry workers, the incidence of pharyngeal gonorrhoea is higher than that of genital tract infection. This may be explained by consistent condom use for vaginal or anal intercourse but not for oral–genital sex.
- Test for rectal gonorrhoea as follows, depending on local clinic and laboratory practices:
  - Obtain material for culture for *N. gonorrhoeae* by gently inserting a cotton wool-tipped applicator stick into the anal canal to a distance of about 2–3 cm, withdrawing, and inoculating a plate of selective culture medium. Or,
  - Obtain material as above and send to the laboratory in appropriate transport medium for culture. Or,
  - if a nucleic acid amplification test (NAAT)[1] is used for the detection of *N. gonorrhoeae*, obtain rectal material using the swab provided by the manufacturers of the test kit, break it into the buffer solution, and send it to the laboratory.

Note: The detection rate of gonococcal infection is identical whether a specimen is obtained blindly or through an anoscope.

The majority of infected women (up to 75% of cases) are symptomless, the remainder having features of a distal proctitis (see Case 20). If she remains untreated, in addition to transmission of

---

[1] Although they are not yet licensed for use on pharyngeal and anorectal specimens, NAATs, particularly single-strand displacements assays (SDA) appear to be more sensitive than culture for the diagnosis of gonorrhoea at these anatomical sites. A positive result in a nucleic acid amplification assay should preferably be confirmed by culture or an alternative NAAT.

infection to a partner, the woman is at risk of complications such as perianal abscess formation and disseminated infection, and she is at increased risk for HIV infection.

- Obtain a specimen of anorectal material for testing for *C. trachomatis* by a NAAT. The swab provided by the manufacturers of the test kit is inserted about 2.5 cm into the anal canal, withdrawn, and the specimen sent in the solution provided to the laboratory. Although these assays are not yet licensed for use on rectal specimens, they are widely used in clinical practice. Most women rectally infected with the common, oculogenital genotypes of *C. trachomatis* are symptomless.
- A serum sample should be tested for hepatitis B surface antigen and core antibody, and if these tests are negative she should be offered vaccination. Several studies have shown that female sex industry workers are at increased risk for this infection. Many health-care providers administer the first dose of vaccine before the results of serological tests are available. Although there is no clear evidence that female sex industry workers are at increased risk of hepatitis A, many physicians vaccinate these women against both hepatitis A and B.
- Serological testing for hepatitis C virus (HCV) infection should be offered. Some, but by no means all, studies have shown an increased prevalence of HCV infection among non-drug-injecting female sex industry workers.

One week later Mary is given the results of the most recent tests: there is no evidence of an STI. She is encouraged to use condoms consistently for penetrative sex with her clients, and she is also encouraged to attend the clinic regularly for screening for STIs. As she has no serological evidence of prior infection with hepatitis B (both hepatitis B surface antigen [HBsAg] and anti-core antibody [anti-HBc] assays were negative), she is offered and accepts vaccination against this infection. Table 3.1 indicates the most commonly used vaccination schedules.

Although more than 95% of healthy vaccinees develop protective antibody, it is good practice to test for a satisfactory immune response about 2 months after the final dose of vaccine. Serological testing of Mary at that time showed a concentration of antibody

TABLE 3.1. Vaccination schedules for hepatitis B.

Engerix B® (20 μg/mL) 1 mL by intramuscular
injection given at 0, 7, and 21 days, with a booster at 12 months

OR*

Engerix B® or HBvaxPRO ® (40 μg/mL) 1 mL by intramuscular
injection at 0, 1, month and 6 months

OR

Engerix B®1 mL by intramuscular injection at 0, 2 weeks,
6 weeks, and 12 months

OR

(if Hepatitis A vaccination also indicated)

Twinrix® 1 mL by intramuscular injection at 0, 7, and 21 days,
with a booster at 12 months

OR

Twinrix® 1 mL by intramuscular injection at 0, 1 month, and
6 months

OR

Twinrix® 1 mL by intramuscular injection at 0, 2, 6 weeks, and
12 months.

*against hepatitis B surface antigen (anti-HBs) of 310 mIU/mL.
What information would you give her?*

Mary has had a good immune response to hepatitis B vaccination. Available data suggest that immunity is likely to be lifelong and that further doses of vaccine are unnecessary. Individuals with sub-optimal levels of anti-HBs should be managed as outlined in Table 3.2.

TABLE 3.2. Interpretation of tests for hepatitis B surface antibody (anti-HBs) after completion of a course of vaccine.

Level of anti-HBs	Action
>100 mIU/mL	No further boosters or serological tests for hepatitis B markers required
10–100 mIU/mL	Give a further dose of vaccine and repeat test for anti-HBs 4–6 weeks later (if still poor response consider no further action)
<10 mIU/mL	Give a further dose of vaccine 6 months after the last dose and repeat anti-HBs test 4–6 weeks later. If still partial response, give a further booster and retest 4–6 weeks later. If the level of anti-HBs is still non-protective, do not give further vaccine but advise patient that he/she is susceptible to infection[a].

[a]Non-responders should be informed that they can receive hepatitis B immunoglobulin (HBIG) if they have a (definite) hepatitis exposure in the future.

Case 4
A Gay Man Requesting a Sexual Health Screen

James is a 43-year-old man who attends a Gay Man's Health Clinic and requests screening for sexually transmissible infections.

What History Would You Obtain from James?

As in Case 1, a specific history should be taken to elicit any symptoms that the individual may not have recognized as being those of a sexually transmissible infection (STI). In addition to the questions posed in that Case, he should be asked if he has symptoms suggestive of distal proctitis: anal discharge or streaking of the stool with "slime," anorectal bleeding, perianal pain, constipation, or a feeling of incomplete defecation. He should also be asked if he has a sore throat. Gonococcal infection of the pharynx is usually symptomless, but a few men (and women) complain of sore throat. (Although there is a good correlation between pharyngeal symptoms and fellatio, this is not the case with respect to gonococcal infection).

A detailed sexual history should then be obtained so that a risk assessment for STIs can be made, and so that the appropriate microbiological tests can be offered.

The history should follow that described in Case 1. In addition:

- Has he ever had anal intercourse, and if so, did he have insertive or receptive intercourse, or both? If he has had anal intercourse, was there consistent condom use? When was the last time, if ever, that he had unprotected anal intercourse?
- Are condoms are always used during oral–genital sex? As oral–genital sexual contact is almost universal among MSM, it is not usually necessary as to make specific enquiry about this activity.

A. McMillan, *Sexually Transmissible Infections in Clinical Practice*, 27
DOI 10.1007/978-1-84882-557-4_4,
© Springer-Verlag London Limited 2009

- Has he been treated previously for syphilis? In many industrialized countries this infection is more prevalent among men who have sex with men (MSM) than among men who have sex with women (MSW). The accurate interpretation of serological tests for syphilis depends on obtaining a good past history (see Cases 18, 19, and 34).
- Has he ever had hepatitis A or B virus infections, or has he been vaccinated against these viruses? Hepatitis B virus (HBV) infection is more prevalent among MSM in geographical areas where the infection is not endemic (see Case 32), and there have been outbreaks of acute hepatitis A among MSM in various countries.

James is symptomless. His last sexual contact had been 3 days previously with the partner with whom he has been in a relationship for 5 years. He has unprotected insertive and receptive oral and anal sex. Both he and his partner had had an HIV antibody test shortly after they had begun the relationship; neither was HIV infected. James has had over 100 lifetime male partners. He has had four casual sexual contacts within the preceding 3 months, the most recent having been 2 weeks previously. Although he does not have genital–anal sex with these casual partners, he does have unprotected receptive and insertive oral–genital and oral–anal contact. He knows that his regular partner also has casual sexual contacts. Most of his partners have been Caucasian, mostly from the United Kingdom or Western Europe, but he is unaware of the country of origin of the other men. He was treated for urethral gonorrhoea when he was 19 years old, but he gives no history of syphilis, hepatitis A, or hepatitis B. He has not been vaccinated against hepatitis A or B. His general health is good, and other than acute appendicitis when he was a young man, he has had no significant past medical problems. He is not currently receiving any medication. Neither he nor, to his knowledge, any of his partners have injected recreational drugs. He uses "poppers" (inhaled alkyl nitrites) to facilitate receptive anal intercourse.

Outline the Physical Examination You Would Perform and Indicate Which Microbiological Tests You Would Undertake in This Case

The physical examination should follow that described for the heterosexual man (Case 1). However, there are additional considerations:

- Take material from the pharynx for culture or for a nucleic acid amplification assay (NAAT) (but see Note 1 in Case 3) for *Neisseria gonorrhoeae* (see Case 3 for details). Pharyngeal gonorrhoea is common among MSM (Fig. 4.1).
- With the patient lying in the left lateral position, examine the perianal region for lesions such as warts (Fig. 4.2 and see Case 15).

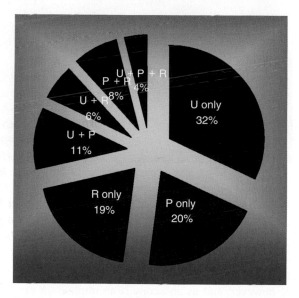

FIGURE 4.1. Anatomical sites of gonococcal infection in 155 MSM. U = urethra; P = pharynx; R = anorectum.

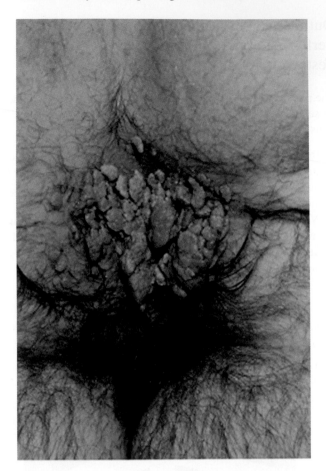

FIGURE 4.2. Perianal warts (condylomata acuminata).

Some clinicians pass an anoscope and examine the anal canal, to diagnose or exclude conditions such as warts, and the distal rectum for signs of proctitis. Few conditions are identified in symptomless patients, however, and as anoscopy is an unpleasant examination for many men, this examination is often omitted. As the anorectum in a common anatomical site of gonococcal and chlamydial infections among MSM (Figs. 4.1 and 4.3), and as receptive anal

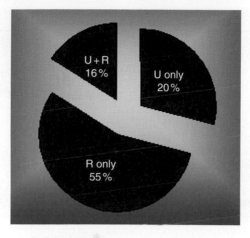

FIGURE 4.3. Anatomical sites of chlamydial infection in 155 MSM. U = urethra; R = anorectum.

intercourse may not be the only means of their acquisition, specimens for the detection of gonococcal and chlamydial infections should always be taken:

- Rectal gonorrhoea is diagnosed or excluded as described in Case 3.
- Rectal chlamydial infection is diagnosed or excluded using a NAAT (see Case 3).
- Offer serological testing for

   ○ Syphilis.
   ○ HIV infection. HIV antibody testing of MSM should be actively encouraged. Early identification of infection results in better health care, and there is evidence that sexual risk-taking is reduced when an individual is known to be HIV infected. Post-exposure prophylaxis can also be made available to serodiscordant couples.
   ○ Current or past HBV infection.
   ○ Previous infection with HAV (the laboratory staff should be asked to test for anti-HAV IgG).
   ○ Hepatitis C virus (HCV) infection. This is an uncommon infection among MSM who do not inject illicit drugs. There

TABLE 4.1. Results of laboratory tests.

Urethral, pharyngeal, and rectal cultures for *N. gonorrhoeae:*
  NEGATIVE.
Testing of urine and rectal material by NAAT for *C. trachomatis*:
  NEGATIVE.
Enzyme immunoassay for treponemal infection: NEGATIVE.
Hepatitis A:
  Anti-HAV IgG: POSITIVE; anti-HAV IgM: NEGATIVE.
Hepatitis B:
  Hepatitis B surface antigen (HBsAg): NEGATIVE
  Anti-hepatitis B core (anti-HBc): POSITIVE
  Anti-hepatitis B surface antigen (anti-HBs): POSITIVE
Hepatitis C:
  Anti-HCV: NEGATIVE

is evidence of an association between "fisting" (the insertion of a clenched fist into the rectum) and HCV infection.

James is offered and accepts vaccination against hepatitis A and B (for vaccination schedule see Case 3), and he is given the first dose of combined vaccine before he leaves the clinic. He is also counseled about safer sexual practices and he is encouraged to use condoms for anal sex with his partner. He is also encouraged to use condoms for oral–genital sex with casual partners and to use a "dental dam" (a square of latex) for oral–anal sex to reduce the risk of acquisition of intestinal pathogens (see Case 31).

James returns the next day and is given a negative HIV antibody test result.

He re-attends the clinic 1 week later to obtain the results of the various tests that had been undertaken (Table 4.1).

How Do You Interpret the Hepatitis A and B Serology Results?

James has been infected previously with HAV. Most acute infections acquired in childhood are symptomless, but about 80% of acute infections in adults are symptomatic. In acute hepatitis A infection, anti-HAV IgM is detectable in the serum; a positive IgG assay indicates previous exposure to the virus. Unlike hepatitis B and C, there is no persistent carrier state.

James has also been infected previously with HBV but has cleared the infection. This is indicated by the negative HBsAg and the positive anti-HBc (and anti-HBs). If the anti-HBc test had been negative, and the anti-HBs test positive, previous vaccination or a false positive anti-HBs would be possible explanations. The majority of acute HBV infections are symptomless, and more than 90% of individuals clear the virus spontaneously. Other persons become persistent carriers (see Case 32), and at risk of the complications of hepatic cirrhosis and hepatocellular carcinoma.

In view of the laboratory findings, it is unnecessary to continue the course of vaccination against either hepatitis A or B.

Case 5
A Man with Urethral
Discharge (1)

*Peter, 19-year-old man, attends you as his General Practitioner 3
days after he had noticed some pain on passing urine and a "moist-
ness" at the tip of his penis.*

What Additional History Would You Elicit?

The history is strongly suggestive of urethritis, and in a young
man, this is usually caused by a sexually transmitted infection. It
is therefore important to take a careful sexual history, as described
in Case 1.

Although urinary tract infections in young men are uncommon,
it is important to ask about other features that may indicate such
infection. For example, has he had frequency, nocturia, urgency, or
lower abdominal pain?

*He tells you that his most recent sexual contact had been 4 days
previously with a young Scottish woman with whom he has been in
a sexual relationship for about 1 month. She is using the combined
oral contraceptive pill as contraception, and he does not use condoms. He tells you that his partner is symptomless. He has had no
other sexual contacts in the preceding 9 months. There is no history of frequency of micturition, nocturia, urgency, or suprapubic
pain.*

What Do You Do Next?

The history suggests that he may have acquired a sexually transmitted infection (STI), for example, *Chlamydia trachomatis* or

A. McMillan, *Sexually Transmissible Infections in Clinical Practice*,   35
DOI 10.1007/978-1-84882-557-4_5,
© Springer-Verlag London Limited 2009

N. gonorrhoeae, or both. The lack of symptoms in his partner is no indication that she does not have a genital tract infection. A consideration of the character of the urethral discharge *may* give a clue to the diagnosis. The majority of men with gonococcal urethritis have a frankly purulent discharge, whereas non-gonococcal urethritis (NGU) tends to be associated with a scant mucoid discharge. Sometimes, however, the discharge associated with urethral gonorrhoea is scant and that of NGU is profuse. Symptoms therefore may not be entirely helpful in differentiating gonococcal from non-gonococcal urethritis. The interval between the sexual contact and the development of symptoms again *may* give an indication of the most likely cause of urethritis – gonorrhoea has a pre-patent period of between 2 and 10 days, whereas that of chlamydial infection tends to be longer (7 days to 5 weeks). There is considerable overlap, however, and in any case Peter has had repeated sexual contact with the same partner over a 1-month period.

The preferred course of action in this case is to refer the patient to the local Sexual Health clinic where there are facilities for rapid diagnosis.

Peter Attends the Clinic. What Do You, as a Sexual Health Specialist Do Next?

It is, of course, essential to confirm the history that was given to Peter's GP.

The next step is to undertake a physical examination. The abdomen is inspected and palpated. The external genitalia are examined as described in Case 1.

There is no abdominal tenderness or guarding, and the kidneys are not palpable. The inguinal lymph nodes are neither enlarged nor tender. Both testes and epididymes are of normal size and consistency, and there is no tenderness. The skin of the shaft of the penis and the glans appear normal. There is a mucoid discharge from the urethra (Fig. 5.1), but neither warts nor ulceration is noted within the meatus.

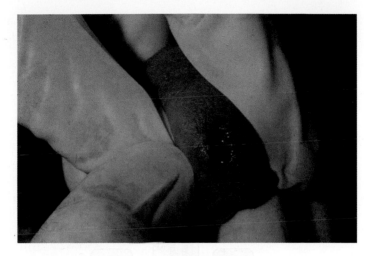

FIGURE 5.1. Mucoid urethral discharge.

What Investigations Would You Undertake?

Material for microscopical examination is obtained by inserting a plastic disposable inoculating loop (10 μL) into the urethra to a distance of about 2–3 cm, gently scraping the walls of the urethra, and withdrawing the loop. A smear is made on a microscope slide, stained by Gram's method, and examined microscopically. Specimens for the detection of gonococcal and chlamydial infections are taken, and screening syphilis and HIV is offered (see Case 1).

You find an average of 20 polymorphonuclear leucocytes in the 10 microscopic fields that you inspected with the oil immersion lens (magnification ×1000). You do not see Gram-negative diplococci.

What is the Probable Diagnosis, and What is the Most Likely Causative Organism?

When more than five polymorphonuclear leucocytes are seen in two of five unselected microscopical fields (×1000 magnification),

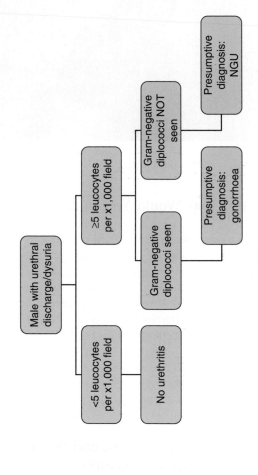

FIGURE 5.2. Diagnosis of urethritis as judged by microscopy.

TABLE 5.1. Causes of non-gonococcal urethritis.

Chlamydia trachomatis	*Ureaplasma urealyticum* [a]
	Mycoplasma genitalium
	Trichomonas vaginalis [b]
	Herpes simplex virus[c]
	Adenoviruses[c]
	Candida spp.[c]
	Trauma[c]

[a]Role in etiology of non-gonococcal, non-chlamydial urethritis not settled.
[b]Uncertainty about the proportion of cases caused by this protozoan, but may be up to 20%.
[c]Uncommon (<1% of cases).

the patient is considered to have urethritis. In the absence of Gram-negative diplococci, the probable diagnosis is non-gonococcal urethritis (NGU) (see Fig. 5.2). (When the smear is unequivocally negative, as in this case, culture for *N. gonorrhoeae* is also negative in at least 95% of cases).

Up to 60% of cases of NGU are caused by *C. trachomatis*. The cause in the others is still uncertain, but Table 5.1 indicates some possible causes. *Mycoplasma genitalium* may cause a proportion of cases (possibly up to 20%); few clinics, however, test routinely for this infection. In a sizeable proportion of NGU cases, an organismal cause cannot be identified.

What Is Your Next Step in Management?

The results of the laboratory tests for *N. gonorrhoeae* and *C. trachomatis* are likely to be unavailable for up to 1 week, and it would be clearly unethical to withhold treatment until they are received. Treatment of chlamydial and non-chlamydial NGU is similar (Table 5.2, but see also Case 22). Azithromycin and doxycycline are equally efficacious in the treatment of chlamydial infection, with cure rates of >95%. Resistance of *C. trachomatis* to tetracyclines and the macrolides is rare. In many clinics

TABLE 5.2. Treatment regimens for uncomplicated anogenital chlamydial infection and non-gonococcal urethritis.

Antimicrobial agent	Dosage
Azithromycin	1 g as a single oral dose[a]
OR	
Doxycycline	100 mg by mouth twice daily for 7 days
OR	
Erythromycin base	500 mg by mouth twice daily for 10–14 days
OR	
Ofloxacin	400 mg by mouth once daily for 7 days

[a]If the patient has eaten within the preceding 2 hours, administration of azithromycin capsules should be delayed. Alternatively, the drug can be given as a suspension in water.

azithromycin is the treatment of choice. It is given under supervision in the clinic, thereby obviating difficulties with adherence. Ofloxacin has similar efficacy to doxycycline, but it is more expensive. Studies have shown that treatment with erythromycin is less effective than the other treatment regimens, and side effects, particularly gastro-intestinal, are common, resulting in difficulties with adherence.

You Opt to Give Him a Single Oral Dose of Azithromycin. What Else Do You Do?

Partner notification is essential and should be undertaken even when *C. trachomatis* is not detected (occasionally the infection may not be identified even when molecular methods of diagnosis are used). In the case of symptomatic men, as was so in Peter, an arbitrary cut-off period of 4 weeks is used to identify those sexual partners potentially at risk. (In symptomless individuals with chlamydial infection, an arbitrary cut-off of 6 months, or until the last sexual partner [whichever is the longer time period] is used). He is advised to abstain from vaginal, oral, and anal intercourse for 7 days after he and his partner have completed treatment. He is asked to contact a clinic nurse in 1 week's time to discuss the results of his tests. At this time it is ensured that treatment has been well tolerated, and that he has not been at risk of re-infection.

Chlamydia trachomatis *was identified in the urine specimen. N.* gonorrhoeae *was not detected in urethral material from Peter and serological tests for syphilis and for HIV yielded negative results. He had no adverse effects of treatment, and he has not had sexual contact in the preceding week.*

Would You Offer a Test of Cure?

A test of cure following treatment for chlamydial infection is not generally undertaken, unless:

- There had been vomiting shortly after ingestion of the azithromycin, or diarrhea had developed within a few hours of dosing.
- There was a possibility of re-infection.
- In the case of a woman, she is pregnant.
- Patient requests.

As specific DNA remains detectable for several weeks after the organism is no longer viable, a test of cure has to be postponed for at least 5 weeks after completion of therapy.

What Are the Complications of Untreated Urethral Chlamydial Infection in a Man?

- Acute epididymitis complicates an indeterminate proportion of men (see Case 13).
- Acute conjunctivitis may result from auto-inoculation from the genital tract.
- Reactive arthritis is a complication in just under 0.5% of cases (see Case 24).

Case 6
A Female Contact of a Man with Presumed Non-gonococcal Urethritis

Anne, Peter's partner (Case 5), *attends the clinic the day following Peter's consultation. She is symptomless and she has had no other sexual contacts during her relationship with Peter. However, she had unprotected vaginal intercourse with an ex-boyfriend a week before beginning the relationship with Peter. Her last menstrual period was been 1 week previously.*

The majority of women – at least 70% – with uncomplicated chlamydial infection are symptomless. In other cases, increased vaginal discharge with or without dysuria, post-coital bleeding, inter-menstrual bleeding, and lower abdominal pain may be features.

She is encouraged to have and accepts screening for sexually transmitted infections (STIs) (see Case 2).

She is certainly at risk of STIs, having had unprotected intercourse with several different and unknown partners. Failure to detect Gram-negative diplococci in a Gram-stained smear of urethral material from Peter, and the subsequent failure to culture *Neisseria gonorrhoeae* from his urethra does not necessarily indicate lack of such infection Anne.

There are no abnormal findings on the external genitalia, perineum, or perianal region. The vagina appears healthy, but there is an edematous, friable ectropion with a mucopurulent discharge from the endocervical canal (Fig. 6.1).

About one-third of women with chlamydial infection have a mucopurulent discharge from the endocervical canal, often with

A. McMillan, *Sexually Transmissible Infections in Clinical Practice*, 43
DOI 10.1007/978-1-84882-557-4_6,
© Springer-Verlag London Limited 2009

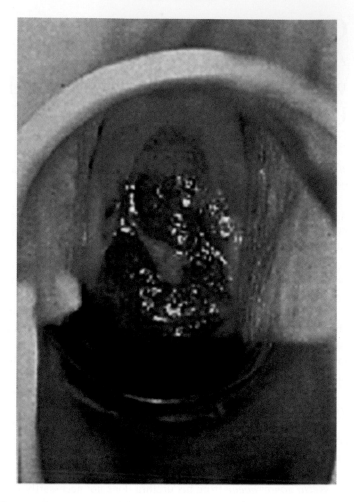

FIGURE 6.1. Ectropion with mucopurulent discharge.

an area of ectopy[1] that is edematous and bleeds easily, as in this case. These changes are not specific, however, and other conditions

---

[1] Cervical ectopy or ectropion refers to a red area of the vaginal cervix, sharply demarcated from the larger area of pink epithelium. The thin columnar epithelium of the endocervical canal is everted, and the area

such as gonococcal infection, endometritis, and salpingitis need to be considered in the differential diagnosis.

What Is the Natural History of Chlamydial Infection in Women in a Woman?

The natural history of genital chlamydial infection is incompletely understood. It is likely that many infections are self-limiting, but, in some women there is evidence for persistence of infection for years. Infected women are at risk of complications:

- Endometritis, salpingitis, and inflammation of the supporting structures of the uterus (pelvic inflammatory disease [PID]) (see Case 14). Although it is difficult to estimate the incidence of PID among infected women, some studies have suggested that between 10 and 40% develop this complication.
- Perihepatitis. Organisms ascend along the peritoneal gutters to infect the liver. There is inflammation of the liver capsule but only superficial hepatitis (see Case 27).
- Bartholinitis (inflammation of the greater vestibular glands that lie in the posterior half of the labia majora and whose orifice is at the junction of the junction of the anterior two-thirds and posterior one-third of the medial aspect of the labia minora).
- Reactive arthritis. This is an uncommon complication affecting <0.5% of women. It is more frequently encountered in males (see Case 24).
- Conjunctivitis. Chlamydial conjunctivitis in both men and women results from auto-inoculation from the genital tract.

What Is Your Immediate Management of This Case?

It is customary to offer treatment to a known contact of an individual with non-gonococcal urethritis, the most common cause of

---

appears red because of the proximity of the blood vessels to the surface. The thick squamous epithelium of the vaginal cervix, however, largely conceals the vessels and hence it appears pink.

which is *Chlamydia trachomatis*. The reasons for this are four-fold:

1) Most chlamydial infections in women are symptomless.
2) If indeed he has chlamydial infection, there is a high probability that she is infected. It is estimated that within sexual relationships the frequency of male–female and female–male transmission is about 70%.
3) Although the sensitivity of the nucleic acid amplification tests (NAATs) is high (see Case 2), occasionally false-negative results are obtained. Discordance between partners in the detection of chlamydiae is recognized.
4) Early studies, before the introduction of NAATs for the diagnosis of chlamydial infection, showed that failure to treat the female partner of a man with non-gonococcal urethritis was more likely to result in recurrence of urethritis when intercourse resumed than if she had been treated.

If she opts to await the results of testing before treatment, then she should abstain from vaginal, oral, and anal intercourse until a negative result is received. If the test is positive, partner notification should be instituted as described in Case 5.

The treatment of contacts follows that described for chlamydial infection in Case 5.

She is offered and accepts treatment with a single oral dose of azithromycin at this initial clinic attendance. Abstention from sexual intercourse, including oral sex, for 7 days is advised.

As advised she telephones a clinic nurse about 1 week later to obtain the results of the laboratory tests: C. trachomatis *was detected in endocervical material, but the other tests were negative. She tells the clinic nurse she had had no side effects from the medication, in particular she had not vomited or had diarrhea immediately after taking the capsules. She also tells the nurse that she has not had any sexual contact since treatment.*

Vomiting and/or diarrhea within 2 hours of taking azithromycin may impair absorption of azithromycin, leading to sub-optimal drug concentrations in the tissues. Re-treatment or a test of cure should be considered under these circumstances.

What Action Would You Take With Respect to Her Ex-boyfriend?

It is possible that this man has been the source of Anne's infection, and he should be advised to seek testing and treatment. Partner notification can be achieved by three means:

- *Patient referral:* The index case informs the sexual partner(s) of the possibility of infection and the need to seek advice from a health-care professional.
- *Provider referral:* Sometimes the index patient is reluctant to contact a sexual partner. In such cases, it is possible, with the patient's consent, for the health-care provider to contact the sexual partner(s), provided there this/these person(s) are identifiable.
- *Conditional referral:* The patient is asked to contact the partner, but if that individual does not seek testing and/or treatment within a reasonable time, say, 3 weeks, the healthcare provider will contact that/these individual(s).

Three days later, Anne telephones the Health Adviser in the clinic, and informs her that the ex-partner is symptomless and will not attend the clinic.

Under These Circumstances, What Possible Action can be Taken?

There is no place for compulsion in securing the clinic attendance of a sexual contact of an individual with an STI. Options include the following:

- Providing the index patient with a single oral dose of azithromycin to give to the person. Although there are several drawbacks to this approach:

  - The inability to ascertain a history of drug allergy,
  - Lack of knowledge about concurrent medication that may interact with the chlamydia therapy,

- Lack of knowledge about any intercurrent medical condition, and, importantly,
- The inability to assess a person's risk of STIs and to promote good sexual health.

Notwithstanding these concerns, several studies have shown that this approach reaches individuals who would not otherwise have been treated and would have continued to pose a public health threat.

Other, innovative, methods of ensuring treatment of chlamydial infection have been devised, including provision of therapy by pharmacists to individuals with documented proof of infection.

Case 7
Urethral Discharge (2)

Richard, who had been married for 2 years, attends a Sexual Health clinic. For the preceding 2 days he has noticed pain on passing urine and a yellow discharge from the tip of his penis. He has no other symptoms.

How Would You Manage His Case?

A careful sexual history should be taken as detailed in Case 1.

For the past 3 months Richard has been working in Eastern Europe, and he returned home 1 week previously. He had unprotected vaginal and oral–genital intercourse with a friend, Maria, 3 days after his return to London, and he had sexual intercourse with his wife 2 days later. As they wish to start a family, he does not use condoms. He has had no other sexual contacts since he married 7 years previously.

The history is that of urethritis and the short interval between sexual intercourse and the onset of symptoms strongly suggests that he has urethral gonorrhoea. There is, however, considerable overlap between the pre-patent periods of gonorrhoea and non-gonococcal urethritis (see Case 5). Physical examination with the taking of the appropriate microbiological tests for gonococcal and chlamydial infections is essential. In addition, he should be offered testing for syphilis and HIV infection, with repeat testing 3 months later if these tests are negative.

When you examine him you note a copious yellow urethral discharge (Fig. 7.1), but there are no other abnormal signs.

A Gram-stained smear of urethral material, taken as described in Case 5, is examined microscopically (Fig. 7.2).

A. McMillan, *Sexually Transmissible Infections in Clinical Practice*,   49
DOI 10.1007/978-1-84882-557-4_7,
© Springer-Verlag London Limited 2009

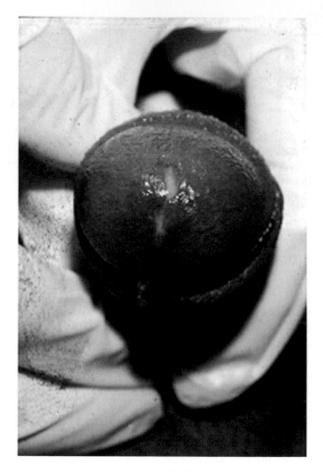

FIGURE 7.1. Mucopurulent urethral discharge.

What Do You See, and What Is the Most Likely Diagnosis?

There are polymorphonuclear leucocytes in this microscopical field, and within the cytoplasm of two of them are Gram-negative diplococci (kidney bean-shaped organisms). The most likely diagnosis then is gonorrhoea, but as other species of *Neisseriae*,

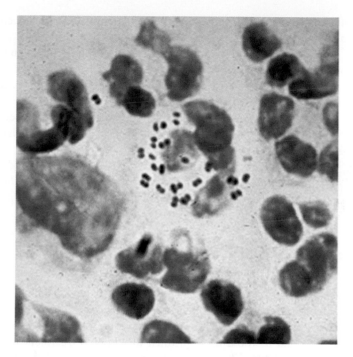

FIGURE 7.2. Gram-stained smear of urethral exudate.

for example, *N. meningitidis*, can colonize the genital tract and are indistinguishable microscopically, culture with the appropriate confirmation of the identity of the isolate is essential.

What Do You Do Next?

Richard is given the presumptive diagnosis of gonorrhoea and consideration is given to the choice of appropriate antimicrobial therapy. Before treatment, however, a throat swab should be taken for culture for *N. gonorrhoeae*. (Pharyngeal gonorrhoea is usually symptomless and it is more difficult to cure than anogenital infection. It is therefore important to identify infection at this anatomical site so that tests can be undertaken to ensure cure. Otherwise the individual may infect or re-infect a sexual partner, and, him/herself be at risk, albeit rarely, of disseminated gonococcal infection).

In choosing the antimicrobial, consideration should be given to the following:

Does he have a history of drug hypersensitivity, and if so, to what agents.

The geographical region where infection was likely to have been acquired, and whether his partner was a local inhabitant or had been visiting from another country.

In Richard's case, he has no known drug allergies. His friend is Philippine and had traveled the week previously from the Philippines to attend a conference in London.

How Does This Knowledge Influence Your Management?

Ideally the treatment used should be based on the results of antibiotic susceptibility tests. These tests, however, take some days to complete and it would be unjustified to withhold treatment until they are available. The choice of drug therefore is dictated by knowledge of the pattern of the sensitivity to antimicrobial agents observed among the strains of the organism in the population of the place of residence of the infecting partner. In this case it has been considered likely that his infection has been acquired from his Philippine friend. In the Far East, including the Philippines, the prevalence of resistance to penicillins, tetracyclines, and the quinolones such as ciprofloxacin is high.

A course of treatment with almost any antimicrobial drug to which the organism is sensitive will cure the majority of patients with gonorrhoea. Patient adherence, however, is often unsatisfactory and tablets may be inadvisably shared with a partner. Strains of organisms with increased resistance to antimicrobials may emerge when courses of treatment prescribed are not completed. For these reasons a single large dose of antibiotic, given under supervision either orally or parenterally, is preferred as treatment of uncomplicated infection. In most cases blood and tissue concentrations of drug reach a high level and are maintained

TABLE 7.1. Regimens currently recommended for the treatment for uncomplicated anogenital gonorrhoea.

Ceftriaxone 250 mg as a single intramuscular injection

OR

Cefixime 400 mg as a single oral dose

OR

Cefotaxime 500 mg as a single intramuscular injection

OR

Spectinomycin 2 g as a single intramuscular injection

for sufficient time to eradicate the organism. Oral administration of antibiotic is preferred to intramuscular injections, which are not only painful but more liable to cause hypersensitivity reactions. Table 7.1 shows some of the more common regimens of treatment of uncomplicated gonorrhoea. With the exception of spectinomycin, these regimens are usually successful in the treatment of pharyngeal infection.

Alternative regimens that can be used when the sensitivity of the infecting organism is known or when the infection has been acquired in a geographical region where the prevalence of resistance is <5% are shown in Table 7.2.

TABLE 7.2. Alternative regimens for the treatment of uncomplicated gonorrhoea.

Amoxicillin 3 g as a single oral dose, plus probenecid 1 g as a single oral dose

OR

Ciprofloxacin 500 mg as a single oral dose

OR

Ofloxacin 400 mg as a single oral dose

The treatment of choice in Richard's case would be a third-generation cephalosporin, and indeed he was given a single oral dose of cefixime.

What Other Treatment Would You Consider?

About 30% of men with gonorrhoea have concomitant infection with *C. trachomatis*. As the cephalosporins are ineffective in the treatment of chlamydiae, concurrent therapy (azithromycin 1 g as a single oral dose) is given to Richard. (Although a first-voided specimen of urine is obtained from Richard for the detection of chlamydiae, the results are not immediately available, and empirical therapy reduces the frequency of follow-up clinic attendances).

What Else Would You Do?

Verbal and written information about gonorrhoea should be provided. Richard should be advised to avoid unprotected sexual contact until he and his partners have completed treatment. Partner notification (contact tracing) is essential in the control of sexually transmitted infections. Consideration should also be given to testing for hepatitis B infection, with the offer of vaccination against this infection if he is not already immune[1] (see Case 3).

A Health Adviser within the clinic interviews Richard. Details are obtained about his recent sexual contacts, and he is encouraged to persuade both his wife and Maria to attend for screening for infection and treatment.

Richard has little difficulty in arranging to contact Maria who is still in the United Kingdom. However, he is guilt-ridden that he may have transmitted an infection to his wife, and he is fearful about the future of his marriage should she learn that he has had extramarital sex. He is therefore reluctant to ask his wife to attend the clinic, but asks about the possibility of being given antibiotics to treat his wife surreptitiously.

---

[1]The prevalence of hepatitis B infection is high (>5% of the population) in South-East Asia, including the Philippines.

What Advice Do You Give, and How Would You Persuade Him to Get His Wife to Attend the Clinic?

It is not routine clinical practice in the management of gonorrhoeae to give antibiotics to a patient about whom you have no knowledge.[2] For example, does she have hypersensitivity to any of the antimicrobial agents that might be prescribed? Is she pregnant? It would also be important to identify complications that often require more prolonged therapy. You therefore decline to prescribe antibiotics for his wife.

When you talk with Richard, you emphasize that confidentiality is paramount in the practice of genitourinary medicine and that the staff will not divulge any information about his infection or about his sexual contact. You do, however, make it clear that should infection be identified in his wife she has the right to know the nature of that infection. It would be entirely wrong for staff to withhold such information.

The symptomless nature of uncomplicated gonorrhoea and chlamydial infection in women is discussed, and the serious sequelae of untreated infection, including pelvic inflammatory disease and disseminated infection, are stressed.

What Is Your Next Course of Action?

It is wise to review Richard 1 week after treatment. At this time

- he should be asked if he has symptoms;
- it should be ascertained whether or not he had had any adverse reaction to the medication;
- importantly, any risk of re-infection should be identified;
- it should be confirmed that partner notification has been completed.

---

[2]An exception may be the treatment of sexual contacts of person with chlamydial infection who can not be persuaded to attend a sexual health clinic (see Case 6).

At the follow-up attendance, Richard is now symptomless, he has not had sexual contact, and he has informed his wife and Maria about the need to attend the clinic. Neisseria gonorrhoeae *had been isolated from the urethra but not from the pharynx. The tests for the other STIs yielded negative results.*

Is a Test of Cure Indicated?

As he is symptomless, as Richard is at follow-up, there is no indication to undertake a test of cure. This, however, should be undertaken if there has been a risk of re-infection, or if pharyngeal gonorrhoea had been identified (in Richard's case, gonococcal infection was not detected in the pharynx). When a test of cure is indicated, this should be performed about a week after completion of therapy, if culture is the diagnostic test, but at least 2 weeks later if a nucleic acid amplification assay is used.

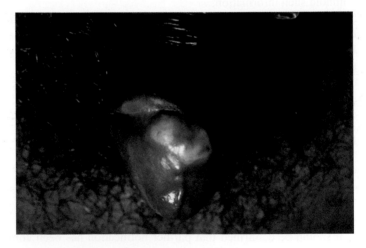

FIGURE 7.3. Gonococcal parafrenal abscess.

What Are the Complications of Untreated Urethral Gonorrhoea in a Man?

- Local complications include abscess formation of the
  - ➢ parafrenal glands (Fig. 7.3);
  - ➢ median raphe;
  - ➢ paraurethral tissues; and rarely,
  - ➢ bulbo-urethral (Cowper's) glands, seminal vesicles, and prostate.
- Acute epididymitis.
- Disseminated infection (see Case 24).
- Acute conjunctivitis from auto-inoculation from the genital tract.

The management of Maria and Richard's wife is discussed in Case 8.

Case 8
A Female Contact of a Man with Gonorrhoea

Richard's partner, Maria, attends the clinic the next day (see Case 7). She is symptomless and was shocked when Richard told her that he had gonorrhoea and that she must have infected him. Her most recent sexual contact had been with Richard, and she had no other sexual partners for 4 months. Her last menstrual period had ended 1 week previously.

What Tests Would You Undertake to Diagnose or Exclude Infection With Neisseria Gonorrhoeae?

Table 8.1 indicates the anatomical sites that may be infected by *N. gonorrhoeae* in a woman.

Maria is examined as described in Case 2. Material is collected from the urethra and endocervical canal for Gram-smear microscopy and culture. Specimens for culture are also collected from the anorectum and pharynx [1] (see Case 3).

There is no apparent urethral discharge and the cervix appears normal. Gram-smear microscopy of urethral and endocervical material fails to identify Gram-negative diplococci.

---

[1]Cure of pharyngeal gonorrhoea is less certain than anogenital infection, and inadequately treated infection at this site may be the source of re-infection of a sexual partner. It is therefore important to recognize pharyngeal gonorrhoea, and undertake at least one test of cure after treatment. Disseminated infection from the pharynx is a recognized complication.

A. McMillan, *Sexually Transmissible Infections in Clinical Practice*, 59
DOI 10.1007/978-1-84882-557-4_8,
© Springer-Verlag London Limited 2009

TABLE 8.1. Anatomical sites that may be infected by *Neisseria gonorrhoeae* in a woman.

Site affected	Frequency of infection at that site *(%)*
Endocervix	85–90
Urethra[a]	65–75
Anorectum[a]	25–50
Oropharynx[a]	5–15

[a]Sole site of infection in ≤5% of women.

What Do You Do?

Many women with gonorrhoea have a mucopurulent discharge from the endocervical canal. As the cervix appears normal in other infected women, absence of infection in this case cannot be inferred from lack of abnormal signs. Although Gram-smear microscopy is helpful in making a presumptive diagnosis of gonorrhoea if Gram-negative diplococci are seen in endocervical or urethral material, the sensitivity of direct microscopy is relatively low: about 50% for endocervical samples and about 20% for female urethral specimens. The negative result in this case therefore does not exclude infection. Culture is more sensitive than direct microscopy, and nucleic acid amplification assays are the most sensitive tests, but, of course, results are not immediately available.

The risk of transmission of *N. gonorrhoeae* from an infected male to a female is estimated to be between 60 and 90%[2]. It is therefore common clinical practice to offer treatment to known sexual contacts of individuals with gonorrhoea before the results of culture or nucleic acid amplification methods are available. If a woman opts to await the results of the microbiological tests before treatment, she is advised to avoid any sexual contact, including oral sex, until negative results are obtained. As the proportion of

---

[2]The risk of a male acquiring gonorrhoea from an infected female is somewhat lower, being estimated to be between 20 and 50%. Studies suggest that inoculum size is important in establishing infection.

infected women detected by culture at their first attendance may be 90% or lower, two sets of investigations need to be taken to diagnose or exclude infection.

As Maria was to return to the Philippines the following day, empirical treatment for gonorrhoea and chlamydial infection[3] was offered and accepted, and she was given oral cefixime as specific treatment for gonorrhoea, and azithromycin for possible chlamydial infection.

Having considered the implications of not informing his wife, Rosemary, that she may have an STI, Richard tells her that his GP thinks that he may have a urinary tract infection and that she should be tested for "infections" and possibly treated with antibiotics. Although Richard tells her that it is best that she should attend the Sexual Health clinic "where they have special facilities to diagnose such urinary infections," he does not divulge the fact that he has already attended.

Several days later, she consults you at the Sexual Health clinic.

How Would You Manage Her Case?

The preservation of a patient's confidentiality is essential, and although you know that Richard probably has gonorrhoea, you must not divulge this fact to his wife without his express consent. In this case, no such consent has been given. A useful opening question is "What has your husband told you?" This allows you to gauge how much he may have told her in the interval between his consultation at the clinic and her attendance.

Rosemary tells you that he has a urinary infection and that the GP has advised that she should attend a specialist clinic. She has had an increased vaginal discharge for about 3 weeks, but had attributed this to stress at work – she is an architect, and has been working long hours at the office to complete an important project. Her most recent menstrual period had begun 10 days before her clinic attendance and had been normal. She uses a combined oral

---

[3]About 40% of women with gonorrhoea have concurrent chlamydial infection.

contraceptive agent and has not missed any pills. When you exam-
ine her you note a mucopurulent discharge from the endocervical
canal. There are no other abnormal findings.

You undertake the tests for the STIs as outlined in Case 2. *Micro-*
scopical examination of a Gram-stained smear of endocervical
material shows many polymorphonuclear leucocytes and intracel-
lular Gram-negative diplococci.

What Would You Do Next?

The presumptive diagnosis is gonorrhoea. However, it would
be unwise to tell her your suspicions at this stage – other
Neisseria species can colonize the genital tract and these are
indistinguishable microscopically from *N. gonorrhoeae*. You tell
her that she may have an infection but that the nature of this can
only be confirmed in the laboratory. You offer and she accepts
empirical treatment before the results of the laboratory tests are
available. She is given cefixime and azithromycin. She is invited to
re-attend the clinic in 7 days.

Rosemary attends the clinic as arranged. Neisseria gonorrhoeae
was cultured from the endocervical canal, urethra, anorectum, and
pharynx. Tests for C. trachomatis *and the other STIs yielded nega-*
tive results.

What Do You Do Next?

It would be improper to withhold the diagnosis from her, and you
tell Rosemary that she has gonorrhoea.

She becomes very agitated and tearful, and asks how and
when she could have acquired this infection. You explain that the
causative organism is sexually transmitted, but it is difficult to
determine its duration. You explore her sexual history further. She
tells you that she had had unprotected sexual intercourse with
a fellow architect, James, about 1 month previously when her
husband had been abroad. Following treatment she has become
symptomless.

As Rosemary had developed symptoms about a week after sex with her colleague, it is possible that he may have been the source of her infection. She is seen by a clinic Health Adviser who persuades her to contact James and suggest that he attend for screening for STIs. She telephones him from the Health Adviser's office. James is angry at the suggestion that he may have an STI and is adamant that he could not have gonorrhoea as neither he nor his wife has symptoms.

Up to about 5% of men with urethral gonorrhoea and the majority of men with pharyngeal infection are symptomless. Although women become infected most commonly from unprotected peno-vaginal intercourse, infection may be acquired through cunnilingus.

As cure of pharyngeal gonorrhoea is less predictable that that of anogenital infection, Rosemary should be offered a test of cure at the follow-up attendance.

What Are the Complications of Untreated Gonorrhoea in a Woman?

- Local complications include inflammation and abscess formation of

  ➢ paraurethral (Skene's) glands;
  ➢ greater vestibular (Bartholin's) glands.

- Pelvic inflammatory disease (see Case 14).
- Disseminated infection and reactive arthritis (see Case 24).
- Acute conjunctivitis from auto-inoculation from the genital tract.

This Case shows how important partner notification is in the control of gonorrhoea and other STIs. It also illustrates that one must not jump to conclusions about the source of these infections.

Case 9
A Woman wih Increased Vaginal Discharge (1)

A 21-year-old woman, Jane, attends you as her General Practitioner because she has noted increased vaginal discharge.

What Points in thc History Would You Wish to Elicit?

Increased vaginal discharge may be physiological, for example, during periods of stress or sexual arousal, or pathological (Table 9.1).

The history can be helpful in the differential diagnosis of increased vaginal discharge. For example, in bacterial vaginosis, the discharge is often described as being white with a fish-like odor that is particularly noticeable after unprotected sexual intercourse. Pruritus vulvae, however, is not a feature of this condition unless there is concurrent infection. The principal symptom of vulvovaginal candidiasis is pruritus vulvae rather than increased vaginal discharge. Jane should therefore be asked about the character of the discharge, any associated odor, and whether or not there is vulval itch. She should be asked if she has been sexually active, and if so the taking of a careful sexual history is important to ascertain her risk of a sexually transmitted infection (see Case 2).

She should, of course, be asked about the date of her last period, if it was of normal duration and character, and her menstrual cycle.

Jane tells you that the discharge is milky in color but there is no abnormal smell after intercourse; she has not had vulval irritation. Her last menstrual period had been about 2 weeks previously, it had occurred at the expected time and had been of usual duration. She has had a boyfriend, Richard, for the past 7 months, and during that time they have been having regular sexual intercourse.

A. McMillan, *Sexually Transmissible Infections in Clinical Practice*, 65
DOI 10.1007/978-1-84882-557-4_9,
© Springer-Verlag London Limited 2009

TABLE 9.1. Causes of a pathological vaginal discharge.		
Vaginal infections	Endocervical infections	Others
Bacterial vaginosis	*Neisseria gonorrhoeae*	Trauma
Trichomonas vaginalis	*Chlamydia trachomatis*	Foreign bodies
Candida spp.		Chemical irritants
Herpes simplex virus		Atrophic vaginitis
Human papillomavirus		Endometritis
		Cervical or vaginal carcinoma

Her partner always uses condoms for vaginal intercourse, but oral sex is unprotected. Richard is Jane's first and only sexual partner.

What is the Most Likely Diagnosis?

The history is strongly suggestive of bacterial vaginosis. One of the symptoms – odor after sexual intercourse – is absent, but this can be explained by the lack of contact of the vaginal secretions with seminal fluid (Richard wears a condom for vaginal intercourse).

You examine Jane, and find a milky-white vaginal discharge that has pooled at the introitus (Fig. 9.1). When you inspect the vaginal

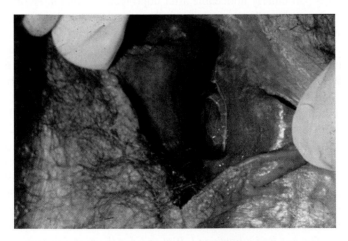

FIGURE 9.1. White discharge at introitus.

walls after having passed a speculum, you note that they are covered with a homogeneous white discharge. The vaginal mucosa, however, does not appear inflamed. The cervix appears normal.

Is Bacterial Vaginosis Still the Most Likely Diagnosis?

The clinical features are characteristic of bacterial vaginosis and suffice to make the diagnosis. The character of the discharge is in keeping with bacterial vaginosis. In trichomoniasis, the discharge is usually yellow-green in color, and in many women the vagina is erythematous and edematous. Occasionally (in less than 5% of women), the cervix shows punctuate hemorrhage sometimes with superficial ulceration – the so-called "strawberry cervix." In women with vaginal candidiasis, the introitus and vagina are often inflamed, and a lumpy, white discharge, often adherent to the vaginal walls, is usually seen.

If You Wished to Clinch the Diagnosis, What Bedside Tests Might You Undertake?

The pH of the vaginal discharge can be measured by smearing some of the discharge on to a strip of narrow-range pH paper (pH 4.0–6.0). The normal pH of vaginal secretions is ≤4.5, but in bacterial vaginosis, it is >5.0. Note that it is important to avoid the alkaline cervical secretions, and the test is invalid in the presence of blood or seminal fluid.

Another test that can be undertaken is the "sniff test." This is performed by suspending some vaginal discharge in a drop of 10% potassium hydroxide on a glass slide held immediately under the nose. An ammoniacal odor can be recognized. The test, however, is subjective and is not recommended in clinical practice.

Note: There is no place for culture of vaginal material in the diagnosis of bacterial vaginosis. The bacteria associated with this condition are constituents of the normal flora, albeit in smaller concentrations. If the diagnosis is to be confirmed, say on account of recurrent symptoms, a specimen of vaginal discharge can be sent to the laboratory in transport medium with instructions to examine a saline-mount preparation and a Gram-stained smear only.

What Would You Expect to See If You Examined Microscopically a Gram-stained Smear of the Discharge?

Lactobacilli that appear as Gram-positive rods predominate in the normal vaginal flora (Fig. 9.2). In bacterial vaginosis, the lactobacilli are reduced in number or are absent, the flora consisting of Gram-positive cocci, Gram-negative rods, and Gram-variable curved rods. These organisms are often found adherent to the surface of epithelial cells (clue cells) (Fig. 9.3).

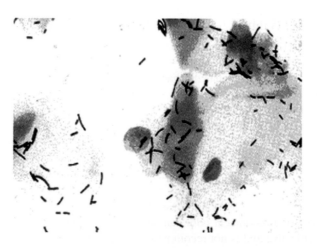

FIGURE 9.2. Lactobacilli.

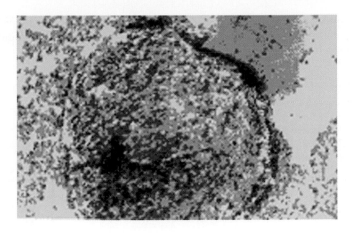

FIGURE 9.3. Bacterial vaginosis – "clue cell."

How Would You Manage Your Patient with Bacterial Vaginosis?

An explanation with written information should be provided. She should be told that it is a common vaginal condition that, for whatever reason, results from overgrowth of organisms that are normally present in the vagina in small concentrations. It is important to stress that it is not a sexually transmitted infection. The underlying cause is still uncertain, but hormonal factors may play a role. Jane should avoid vaginal douching, the use of shower gels and the use of antiseptic lotions in her bath – factors known to be associated with the condition. Table 9.2 shows the antimicrobial drug regimens that are generally available for the treatment of bacterial vaginosis. Metronidazole by mouth, either as a course or in a single dose is the treatment of choice.

Each regimen is very effective. Recurrence, however, is common, and may require further courses of treatment.

Although Jane is in a regular relationship, and has had no other partners, it might be worth offering testing for at least chlamydial infection.

TABLE 9.2. Drug regimens for the treatment of bacterial vaginosis.

Metronidazole 400–500 mg twice daily for 5–7 days[a]
OR
Metronidazole 2 g as a single oral dose[a]
OR
Metronidazole 0.75% gel instilled into the vagina nightly for 7 days
OR
Clindamycin 2% cream instilled into the vagina nightly for 7 days[b]
OR
Clindamycin capsules 300 mg twice daily by mouth for 7 days[c]

[a]Patients must be warned of the interaction between alcohol and metronidazole (see Case 10).
[b]May affect the integrity of latex condoms.
[c]May be associated with antibiotic-associated diarrhea.

How Would You Manage Her Sexual Partner?

There is no evidence that the organisms of bacterial vaginosis are sexually transmitted, and so there is no advantage in treating Richard.

Case 10
Vaginal Discharge (2)

Mary is a 26-year-old woman who attends a Sexual Health clinic. For the preceding 2 weeks she has noticed a profuse, yellow vaginal discharge that has a rather musty smell. She also has noted mild irritation on the vulva and she has had some discomfort on passing urine. She is otherwise symptomless. Her menstrual periods are regular; the most recent began 21 days previously and was of usual character. Her general health is good and there is no past history of any sexually transmissible infections.

You elicit a sexual history as described in Case 2. *Four weeks before she attends you she had returned to the United Kingdom from India where she had taught English in a rural school. She had had unprotected vaginal intercourse with a local man with whom she had had a 2-month relationship. Her most recent sexual contact with him had been 2 days prior to her departure from India.*

What Conditions Would You Consider in the Differential Diagnosis?

The causes of increased vaginal discharge are shown in Table 9.1. Bacterial vaginosis is usually associated with a white vaginal discharge, and unless there is concurrent infection with, for example, *Candida* spp., pruritus vulvae is not a feature. Pruritus vulvae is the cardinal symptom of candidiasis, and as Mary has noticed only mild vulval irritation, this is not the most likely diagnosis. Gonococcal and chlamydial infections can cause increased vaginal discharge and dysuria, but the profuse discharge that Mary describes would be unusual. Trichomoniasis, caused by the

A. McMillan, *Sexually Transmissible Infections in Clinical Practice*,
DOI 10.1007/978-1-84882-557-4_10,
© Springer-Verlag London Limited 2009

flagellated protozoan *Trichomonas vaginalis*, may be associated with an increased yellow vaginal discharge and dysuria. Primary genital herpes usually causes marked vulval pain and dysuria and is therefore an unlikely diagnosis here. The symptoms of recurrent genital herpes, however, are usually less severe and can include vulval irritation and dysuria; the profuse discharge described by Mary would, however, be unusual. The presence of a foreign body such as a retained tampon is often associated with a profuse foul-smelling vaginal discharge, and this needs to be excluded.

When you examine Mary you find that there is marked reddening of the introitus, but there is no ulceration. There is no foreign body in the vagina, but the walls are inflamed and a frothy yellow discharge pools in the posterior fornix.

What Investigations Would You Undertake?

Although the clinical appearance is strongly suggestive of trichomoniasis, this is not pathognomic, and laboratory tests are required to confirm the diagnosis (see Case 2). On microscopy of a wet preparation *Trichomonas vaginalis*, which is larger than a polymorphonuclear leucocyte but smaller than an epithelial cell, is readily recognized by its usually rapidly moving flagella, the rippling movement of the undulating membrane, and the jerky movements of the organism. Ideally the specimen should be examined immediately but if this is impracticable the swab should be placed preferably in transport medium such as Amies'.

Ideally, a vaginal specimen should be sent to the laboratory for culture. Cultivation for *T. vaginalis*, however, is regarded by many as expensive and time consuming, and it is not widely available. The detection of specific DNA by polymerase chain reactions appears to be more sensitive than wet smear microscopy and culture, and nucleic acid amplification tests (NAATs) for the diagnosis of vaginal trichomoniasis are available in some UK clinics.

A Gram-stained smear of vaginal exudate is also prepared for microscopical examination for *Candida* spp. Material from the endocervical canal is obtained for Gram-smear microscopy and culture or NAAT for *Neisseria gonorrhoeae*, and a sample is also obtained for the detection of *Chlamydia trachomatis* (see Case 2).

The urethra should be sampled using a 10 μL plastic inoculating loop for the detection of *N. gonorrhoeae* by Gram-smear microscopy and culture or NAAT.

Syphilis is more prevalent in India than in the United Kingdom, and serological tests, for example, the anti-treponemal enzyme immunoassay, should be undertaken. As the pre-patent period of syphilis is up to 90 days, a further blood sample should be tested 3 months after the most recent sexual contact in India, if the initial test is negative. At least 50% of individuals with infectious syphilis are symptomless and have no signs of infection. These infected persons can only be identified by serological testing.

As the incidence of HIV is increasing in India, it is worth counseling Mary about this infection and the advantages of having an HIV antibody test at an appropriate time (see Case 1).

The saline-mount preparation of vaginal exudate shows T. vaginalis. *When you examine the Gram-stained smear of vaginal material you find many polymorphonuclear leucocytes (Fig. 10.1), lactobacilli are absent, and no fungal hyphae are seen. Gram-negative diplococci suggestive of* Neisseria gonorrhoeae *are not identified in Gram-stained smears from the endocervical canal and urethra.*

As trichomonads cannot be identified reliably in a Gram-stained smear, this is not a useful diagnostic test. Women with trichomoniasis often show similar vaginal pH changes and alteration to the vaginal microflora as found in bacterial vaginosis (see Case 9).

What Treatment Would You Provide, and What Follow-Up Would You Offer?

Metronidazole is the treatment of choice. Recommended treatment regimens for adults are shown in Table 10.1

At the dose generally used for trichomoniasis, metronidazole is well tolerated and during more than 30 years of its widespread use, it has earned a reputation of being remarkably safe. Occasional side effects at these doses include nausea, an unpleasant taste in the mouth, furring of the tongue and gastrointestinal upsets; headache, dizziness, anorexia, depression, and skin eruptions have been reported but rarely.

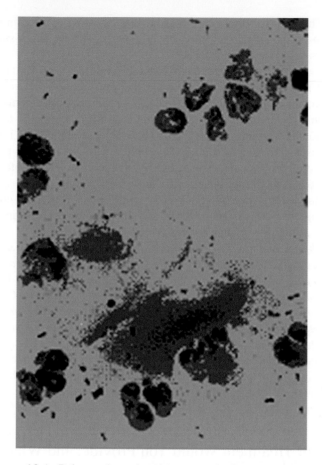

FIGURE 10.1. Polymorphonuclear leucocytes in Gram-stained vaginal smear.

Mild-to-moderate disulfiram-like effects have been described (e.g., facial flushing, headache, nausea, and sweating) with metronidazole, following alcohol ingestion. Adverse effects of concurrent metronidazole and alcohol are infrequent but patients should be advised about these possibilities in the event of alcohol being ingested during metronidazole therapy and for at least 48 h after its completion.

TABLE 10.1. Drug regimens for the treatment of trichomoniasis.

Metronidazole as a single oral dose of 2 g, given either in tablet form (four, 400 mg tablets) and taken during or after a meal or in suspension taken at least 1 h before a meal
OR
Metronidazole 400–500 mg twice daily, during or after a meal, for 5–7 days

There is no evidence that metronidazole is teratogenic or associated with birth defects. It is recommended, however, that high doses of the drug should be avoided in pregnancy.

You arrange to see Mary 1 week later to ensure that treatment has been successful and to provide the results of the other laboratory tests. You also suggest that her partner be treated for trichomoniasis.

What Are the Clinical Features of Trichomoniasis in Men, and How Is the Condition Diagnosed?

About 50% of men with trichomoniasis are symptomless. When there are symptoms, urethral discharge that is usually small to moderate in amount is the most common feature. Frequency of micturition and mild dysuria may also be features. Balanoposthitis, which may rarely be ulcerative, may be associated with. *T. vaginalis* infection.

If a urethral discharge is present, this can be collected with a 10 µL inoculating loop, otherwise a scraping should be taken gently from the urethra before the patient passes the first morning urine. A saline-mount preparation is made as in the female and examined microscopically for *T. vaginalis*. If possible, urethral material should be cultured for the organism, or tested by a NAAT. A centrifuged deposit (600*g*) of a 20 mL urine sample taken preferably after the patient has held his urine overnight may also be examined microscopically, by culture or by a NAAT.

As re-infection of the sexual partner is almost invariable if he is not treated, the man should be given metronidazole, irrespective of the laboratory findings if tests are undertaken (empirical therapy is often given without the undertaking of tests).

When Mary attends for follow-up she states that her vaginal discharge persists. You now have the results of the other laboratory tests. Although Gram-smear microscopy for N. gonorrhoeae *was negative, the organism was cultured from the endocervical canal and urethra.* Chlamydia trachomatis *was also detected in the endocervical canal. Serological tests for syphilis and for HIV were negative. Saline-mount microscopy of vaginal exudate once again shows* T. vaginalis. *You treat the gonococcal and chlamydia infections with the appropriate antimicrobial drugs and arrange the necessary follow-up (see Case 8). She has telephoned her partner in India, and he has sought treatment there.*

The importance of screening for other sexually transmitted infections (STIs) in individuals in whom one is detected is shown in this case. In the past, trichomoniasis was associated with other STIs in up to 40% of women attending sexually transmitted diseases clinics in the United Kingdom during the 1960s.

Treatment failure is more often the result of failure to adhere to the treatment regimen, vomiting of the drug, or re-infection than to drug resistance. Inability to produce trichomonicidal concentrations in vaginal tissue of fluid may contribute to treatment failure. Sometimes persistent infection may result from inactivation of metronidazole by vaginal aerobic and anaerobic bacteria, and treatment with a course of amoxicillin or erythromycin before re-treatment with metronidazole may be effective. Resistance to the 5-nitroimidazoles, of which metronidazole is one such drug, does occur, but facilities to test for susceptibility to these drugs are unavailable outwith a research setting. As metronidazole resistance is relative rather than an all-or-one phenomenon, many women infected with resistant stocks of *T. vaginalis* can be cured by increasing doses of metronidazole. For example, metronidazole can be given in an oral dose of 400 mg three times daily, with the insertion of a 1 g suppository rectally once daily, for at least 7 days. The intravenous route can be used if the woman cannot tolerate the oral formulation. The drug can also be given in a daily oral dose of 2 g for 3–5 days. Alternatively, as this drug may be more active against some stocks of *T. vaginalis*, high doses of tinidazole (2 g daily for 14 days) may affect cure in women with refractory trichomoniasis.

Case 11
Pruritus Vulvae

Margaret is a 25-year-old solicitor who has been married for 5 years, her husband having been her first and only sexual partner. She presents to you as her General Practitioner with a 4-day history of itch in the vulva and a little vaginal discharge. Her general health is good and she has not had similar symptoms before. Her last menstrual period had ended 8 days previously; she uses the combined oral contraceptive pill. She tells you that her husband has had mild itch and redness of his penis, these symptoms developing a few hours after most recent sexual intercourse 2 days previously.

What is the Most Likely Diagnosis?

Pruritus vulvae is the most common symptom in women with candidiasis, and this diagnosis must be high on the list of probabilities. There are, however, other causes of acute pruritus vulvae that you may wish to consider (Table 11.1)

As you do not have a chaperone available, you do not examine Margaret, but you consider the most likely diagnosis to be candidiasis.

What Treatment Do You Offer?

With respect to efficacy in the treatment of acute vulvovaginal candidiasis, there is little difference between the various antifungal drugs and their route of administration. In the selection of an agent, however, several factors should be taken into consideration:

- patient choice between a topical or oral preparation;
- pregnancy, or the possibility of pregnancy at the time of treatment;

A. McMillan, *Sexually Transmissible Infections in Clinical Practice*, DOI 10.1007/978-1-84882-557-4_11, © Springer-Verlag London Limited 2009

TABLE 11.1. Some causes of pruritus vulvae other than candidiasis.

Condition	Comments
Herpes simplex virus infection	*Pain* is the usual feature of primary infection
Trichomoniasis	Vaginal discharge is the most common symptom
Irritant contact dermatitis	Most common irritants are soap and infected vaginal secretions. Patients should be asked about use of possible irritants
Eczema	Secondary infection with *Candida* spp. or less commonly by bacteria may complicate eczema
Allergic contact dermatitis	Usually occurs 1–2 days after exposure to the allergen. Indistinguishable morphologically from irritant contact dermatitis. Allergens include topical antifungal creams and preservatives
Lichen planus	
Psoriasis	Usually lesions elsewhere, e.g., finger nail pitting, scalp lesions.
Lichen sclerosus	
Depression and anxiety	Often exacerbate pruritus
Vulva intraepithelial neoplasia	

- in the case of topical preparations, the possibility of damage to latex condoms or contraceptive diaphragms;
- in the case of oral antifungal drugs, the possibility of drug interactions, although the risk is small with single-dose therapy;
- cost.

Tables 11.2 and 11.3 summarize the available agents. With the possible exception of clotrimazole preparations for which data are lacking, the topical antifungal agents may alter the latex of condoms and contraceptive diaphragms, leading to failure. It is important that the patient is aware of this possibility. Although there is no evidence for any adverse effect in pregnancy, all topical agents

TABLE 11.2. Topical agents for use in acute vulvovaginal candidiasis.

Antifungal agent	Formulation	Dosage
Clotrimazole	Vaginal pessary, containing 500 mg clotrimazole.	One inserted at night for one night
	Vaginal pessary, containing 200 mg clotrimazole,	One inserted nightly for 3 nights
	Vaginal pessary, containing 100 mg clotrimazole	One inserted nightly for 6 nights
	Vaginal cream, containing 10% clotrimazole	5 g inserted at night for one night
Miconazole	Capsule, containing 1200 mg miconazole	One inserted vaginally for one night
	Cream, containing miconazole 2% w/w	5 g inserted nightly for 10–14 days, OR, twice daily for 7 days
Econazole	Vaginal pessary for single-dose use, containing 150 mg econazole	One inserted at night for one night
	Cream, containing econazole 1% w/w	5 g inserted nightly for 14 days
Nystatin	Vaginal tablet containing 100,000 units nystatin	One inserted nightly for 14 nights

TABLE 11.3. Oral antifungal agents for the treatment of acute vulvovaginal candidiasis.

Drug	Dosage
Fluconazole	150 mg capsule as single dose
Itraconazole	Two 100 mg capsules twice daily for 1 day

should be used with caution, and only when the benefits of treatment are likely to outweigh any potential risk. The patient should be fully involved in the discussions. *The oral antifungal drugs should be avoided in the treatment of pregnant women with vulvovaginal candidiasis.*

Margaret opts for treatment with a single clotrimazole pessary.

What Conditions May Pre-dispose to Acute Vulvovaginal Candidiasis?

In the majority of women with acute vulvovaginal candidiasis, there are no obvious predisposing factors; Table 11.4, however, indicates some such factors.

Margaret is informed that if her symptoms do not resolve rapidly that she should re-attend the G.P.

Although the most likely diagnosis is candidiasis, failure to respond to antifungal therapy signals reconsideration of the diagnosis (but see Case 26).

The management of balanoposthitis is discussed in Case 12.

TABLE 11.4. Factors pre-disposing to acute vulvovaginal candidiasis.

Pregnancy
Uncontrolled diabetes mellitus
Immunosuppressive states, e.g., HIV infection
Immunosuppressive drugs, e.g., corticosteroids
Antibiotic use

Case 12
A Man with a Red, Itchy Penis

Michel, a 19-year-old student, attends a Sexual Health clinic with a 2-day history of having an itchy red penis. He is otherwise well, and he is not receiving any medication. There have not been previous episodes of genital inflammation. His first sexual intercourse had been 3 days previously with a young woman whom he had met at a club. He used a condom only toward the end of vaginal intercourse.

There is erythema of the glans penis and the mucosal surface of the prepuce which is mildly edematous with minor fissuring (Fig. 12.1).

What Is This Condition, and What Are Possible Causes?

This is balanoposthitis,[1] a term encompassing a variety of conditions, the appearance of some of which is characteristic.

A common predisposing factor for balanoposthitis is poor hygiene with the accumulation of smegma in the preputial sac. Irritants such as antiseptics, spermicidal lubricants, soap, or shower gels may cause balanoposthitis.

Bacteria, yeasts, or *Trichomonas vaginalis* are recognized infective causes. Edema of the glans and prepuce from such infective causes may result in phimosis, with secondary anaerobic infection producing a malodorous subpreputial discharge sometimes with painful, tender ulceration, and inguinal lymphadenitis. Aerobic

---

[1]The terms balanitis and posthitis refer, respectively, to inflammation of the glans and mucosal surface of the prepuce.

A. McMillan, *Sexually Transmissible Infections in Clinical Practice*, 81
DOI 10.1007/978-1-84882-557-4_12,
© Springer-Verlag London Limited 2009

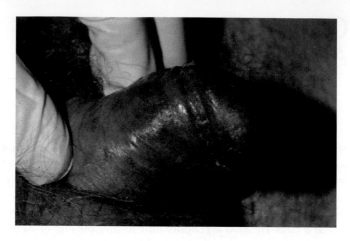

FIGURE 12.1.

infections such as Group B β-hemolytic streptococci and Group A hemolytic streptococci can also cause balanoposthitis.

Characteristic symptoms of candidiasis are soreness and itching of the penis, accompanied sometimes by material collecting under the prepuce. On examination there may be a balanoposthitis with superficial erosions and sometimes eroded maculopapular lesions and preputial edema. There may be fissuring of the prepuce, particularly at its orifice. On occasions there may be a balanoposthitis with erosions without detectable yeasts appearing 6–24 h after intercourse with a partner who has vaginal candidiasis. Such a balanitis may be due to sensitivity to yeast-containing vaginal discharge.

Balanoposthitis, which may rarely be ulcerative, can be caused by *Trichomonas vaginalis*. Herpes simplex virus may be isolated from erosions, and rarely, causes a necrotizing balanitis. Chronic or recurrent balanoposthitis has been associated with human papillomavirus infection.

Balanoposthitis may be a component of a generalized skin disease such as fixed drug eruption or erythema multiforme exudativum and may be associated with diabetes or debilitating disease, particularly in the elderly. Circinate balanitis (psoriasis) may be a feature of sexually acquired reactive arthritis (see Case 24).

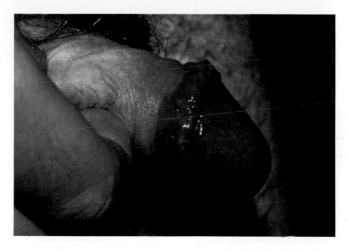

FIGURE 12.2. Plasma cell balanitis.

All forms of balanitis may become chronic or relapse frequently, particularly in the elderly, when fibrotic changes are those seen in lichen sclerosus.

Plasma cell balanitis (of Zoon) (**Fig. 12.2**) is a chronic condition diagnosed in middle-aged or elderly uncircumcised men. There is a localized shiny moist erythematous plaque on the glans penis. Biopsy shows a dense plasma cell infiltration of the dermis.

What Investigations Would You Undertake in This Case?

Bacterial culture can exclude an infective etiology and is sometimes diagnostic. It is also helpful to look for *Candida* species. *As balanoposthitis, particularly candidal, can be the presenting feature of diabetes mellitus, the urine should always be tested for glucose.* Culture of herpes simplex virus from ulcers or erosions should be attempted. When trichomonal infection is suspected, material from the subpreputial sac should be examined microscopically, and, if available, by culture or a nucleic acid amplification assay.

Tests for sexually transmitted infections should be undertaken after the appropriate interval (see Case 1).

Gram-smear microscopy of material collected from the subpreputial sac shows fungal hyphae.

How Would You Treat This Patient, and How Would You Manage the Other Causes of Irritant or Infective Balanoposthitis?

Candidal balanoposthitis is treated with a topical imidazole, or with fluconazole given in a single dose of 150 mg by mouth (see Case 11). The use of an imidazole cream containing 1% hydrocortisone is often used in patients with marked inflammation and preputial edema.

In the management of mild irritant balanoposthitis, the topical application emollients such as Dermol®cream may be helpful. Sensitizing agents such as soaps should not be used during acute inflammation, and emollients can also be used as soap substitutes. Topical hydrocortisone cream 1% w/w applied three times per day for 7 days is often successful in those patients whose irritant balanoposthitis fails to resolve to emollients. When they have been implicated as the cause of the balanoposthitis in the individual, spermicides should be avoided subsequently.

Mild forms of infective balanitis are cleared readily by retracting the prepuce and bathing with physiological saline. This treatment should be repeated twice or thrice daily. The prescription of metronidazole in an oral dosage of 400 mg twice daily by mouth for 7 days is useful in the treatment of anaerobic balanoposthitis. When phimosis is present, subpreputial lavage with saline 3–6 hourly, using a disposable hypodermic syringe is often sufficient to promote drainage and healing.

The management of plasma cell balanitis should only be undertaken by an experienced clinician. Treatment is with a potent topical corticosteroid cream such as clobetasol, with circumcision being indicated when a satisfactory response is not observed after a reasonable interval, of, say 3 months.

Case 13
A Man with Scrotal Pain

*Michael, a 21-year-old man, presents to an Emergency Depart-
ment with a 5 h history of pain and swelling of the left scrotum.
The pain came on gradually and is increasing in severity. He has
not noticed urethral discharge or dysuria, and there has been no
frequency, hesitancy, or urgency of micturition, nocturia, hematuria, or abdominal or loin pain. There is no history of trauma.
His general health is good and he is not receiving any medication.*

What Are the Causes of Acute Scrotal Pain?

Table 13.1 shows some causes of acute scrotal pain.

The history alone can only really exclude trauma as a cause of
his pain.

*The left scrotal skin is reddened (Fig. 13.1). There is tenderness
and swelling of the left epididymis but because of the presence of
a hydrocoele, the testis cannot be palpated. There is a mucoid urethral discharge.*

What Is the Most Likely Diagnosis?

The most likely diagnosis is acute epididymitis, probably associated with chlamydial infection (see Case 5). However, testicular torsion must be excluded. In the typical patient with torsion,
there is a sudden onset of pain in the affected side of the scrotum, sometimes with nausea and vomiting. The testis often lies
more horizontal than usual and is high in the scrotum. The lower
pole of the affected testis is exquisitely tender. When these features
are present, surgical exploration is mandatory. The viability of the

A. McMillan, *Sexually Transmissible Infections in Clinical Practice*,   85
DOI 10.1007/978-1-84882-557-4_13,
© Springer-Verlag London Limited 2009

TABLE 13.1. Some causes of acute scrotal pain.

Acute epididymo-orchitis
Testicular torsion
Trauma
Torsion of the appendix testis or of the epididymis
Hemorrhage or infarction of a testicular tumor
Testicular infarction associated with, for example, autoimmune
    diseases or leukemia

testis that has undergone torsion depends on the degree of torsion
and the duration of symptoms, and surgical intervention should be
undertaken as soon as possible after onset of symptoms. Clinical
signs are not always reliable, but imaging studies may give valuable assistance.

*An ultrasound examination of the scrotum is performed. The epi-
didymis is swollen and hypoechoic but the testis appears normal.*

This finding confirms the clinical diagnosis. It should be noted
that torsion of the testis is not easy to diagnose by real-time scrotal ultrasonography. Color Doppler ultrasound, however, is useful
in differentiating acute torsion from epididymo-orchitis, particularly when sophisticated equipment and "power" Doppler are used.
In torsion, blood flow is either absent or reduced, whereas in
epididymo-orchitis it is increased. Ultrasonography cannot diagnose all cases of torsion – false-negative results do occur – and if
there is doubt about the diagnosis surgical exploration is indicated.

What Are the Causes of Acute
Epididymo-Orchitis?

Table 13.2 lists the causes of epididymo-orchitis.

In young men (under the age of 35 years), epididymitis is usually associated with a sexually transmitted infection, particularly
Chlamydia trachomatis. In industrialized countries where access to
medical care is good, gonococcal epididymo-orchitis is rare. Acute
epididymitis in older men (over 35 years of age) usually occurs
as a result of a complicated urinary tract infection, usually due to
coliform organisms. This does not imply that sexually transmitted

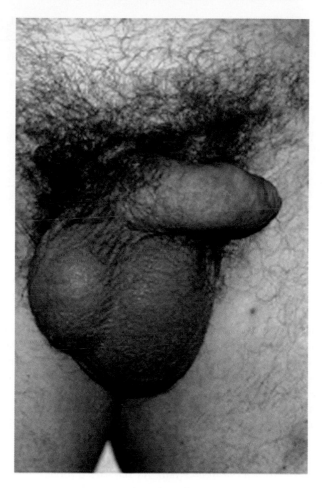

FIGURE 13.1. Left scrotal redness and swelling.

infections do not cause epididymo-orchitis in older men – a sexual history should be elicited. The prevalence of coliform infection in epididymo-orchitis in young men who have sex with men who have had unprotected insertive anal intercourse is higher than in men who have sex with women. As anatomical abnormalities of

TABLE 13.2. Causes of epididymo-orchitis.

Chlamydia trachomatis
Neisseria gonorrhoeae
Urinary tract pathogens, e.g., *Escherichia coli*
Mumps
Amiodarone (used in the treatment of arrhythmias)[a]
Mycobacterium tuberculosis [b]
Mycobacterium leprae [b]
Brucella spp.[b]
Systemic fungal infections, e.g., histoplasmosis[b]
Filariasis[b]

[a]Rare.
[b]Rare in industrialized countries.

the urinary tract are common in men with Gram-negative bacterial infections, especially in those aged 50 years and over, urological investigations are indicated in this group of patients.

In mumps, epididymo-orchitis complicates about 20% of cases in adults, with one in six showing bilateral involvement. Scrotal swelling is usually noted within a week of parotid enlargement, but sometimes only when the clinical signs of mumps have disappeared.

Michael is referred immediately to a Sexual Health clinic.

He has been sexually active for about 3 years and has had four partners in that time. For the past 2 months he has been in a regular sexual relationship with an 18-year-old woman, his only sexual partner for more than 1 year. As she uses a progesterone-only implant for contraception, they do not use condoms for vaginal sex. She is symptomless.

A Gram-stained smear of urethral material shows more than 10 polymorphonuclear leucocytes per ×1,000 microscopical field; Gram-negative diplococci are not identified. Specimens for the detection of chlamydial and gonococcal infections are taken as described in Case 1, *and a mid-stream specimen of urine is sent to the laboratory for culture for urinary tract pathogens. He agrees to serological testing for syphilis and HIV. Treatment is initiated without waiting for the laboratory test results.*

TABLE 13.3. Drug treatment of acute epidiymo-orchitis.

For presumed gonococcal infection:

Ceftriaxone 250 mg as single intramuscular injection
PLUS
Doxycycline 100 mg twice daily by mouth for 10–14 days

For presumed chlamydial infection:

Doxycycline 100 mg twice daily by mouth for 10–14 days

For presumed infection with Gram-negative bacteria:

Ofloxacin 200 mg twice daily by mouth for 14 days
OR
Ciprofloxacin 500 mg twice daily by mouth for 10 days

Table 13.3 shows the currently recommended regimens for the treatment of epididymo-orchitis.

Michael is treated with doxycycline for 14 days. He is also advised to rest and to abstain from sexual intercourse until he and his partner has completed treatment. For analgesia, ibuprofen, a non-steroidal anti-inflammatory drug, is prescribed. Partner notification is also completed during this clinic visit. His girlfriend attends the clinic the next day for screening and empirical treatment with a single oral dose of 1 g of azithromycin.

Michael is reviewed 3 days after initiation of therapy. There has been considerable improvement in his symptoms, and the epididymis is less tender.

The results of the tests taken at the initial attendance are available: a nucleic acid amplification test for C. trachomatis *was positive, but* Neisseria gonorrhoeae *was not detected. Serological tests for syphilis and HIV were negative.*

If There had been no Significant Improvement at This Time, What Conditions Would You Then Consider?

Failure to have improved at this time would have prompted a reassessment of the original diagnosis (Table 13.4).

TABLE 13.4. Conditions that may be associated with failure to respond to antimicrobial drugs in a man with suspected epididymo-orchitis.

Testicular, or rarely, epididymal neoplasm
Testicular ischemia or infarction
Testicular infarction or abscess formation, particularly with
    gonococcal infection or pyocele of the scrotum, as a complication
    of pyogenic bacterial orchitis
Tuberculous epididymo-orchitis
Mumps orchitis
Fungal epididymo-orchitis

When Michael attends the clinic 1 month later he is symptomless. The right epididymis remains swollen and firm but is not tender.

Thickening of the epididymis can persist for several months, and further intervention at this stage is not indicated.

Case 14
A Young Woman with Abdominal Pain (1)

Sarah, an 18-year-old woman, presents to her General Practitioner with a 1-week history of intermittent cramping lower abdominal pain and increased vaginal discharge. She has felt feverish. Her bowel movements have been normal and she has had no urinary symptoms. For the past 4 months she has been in a regular relationship with a young man. They last had sex 3 days previously during which Sarah experienced lower abdominal pain. Her menstrual cycle has always been regular, the last period having been 3 weeks previously and normal. She has, however, noticed intermittent slight vaginal bleeding since then. Condoms are used for contraception, but occasionally, most recently 3 weeks ago, intercourse has been unprotected.

What Conditions Do You Consider in the Differential Diagnosis?

Table 14.1 shows some conditions associated with lower abdominal pain in a young woman.

In a young sexually active woman, pelvic inflammatory disease (PID) or ectopic pregnancy must be considered high on the list of probabilities. In acute appendicitis, the nausea is usually more pronounced, and constipation is a common feature. As the pain is severe and usually of sudden onset, rupture of an ovarian or endometriotic cyst is an unlikely cause. The lack of urinary and gastrointestinal symptoms makes conditions such as cystitis or enteritis, respectively, unlikely.

She looks well and is not in obvious distress. Her temperature is 37.2°C, her pulse is 75 per minute, and her blood pressure is

A. McMillan, *Sexually Transmissible Infections in Clinical Practice*,
DOI 10.1007/978-1-84882-557-4_14,
© Springer-Verlag London Limited 2009

TABLE 14.1. Causes of lower abdominal pain in a young woman.

Ectopic pregnancy
Pelvic inflammatory disease
Acute appendicitis
Ruptured ovarian cyst/follicle
Ovarian torsion
Miscarriage
Urinary tract infection
Urinary calculi
Enteritis

130/75 mmHg. The abdomen moves well with respiration. She has tenderness but no guarding in both iliac fossae. Neither liver nor spleen is palpable. Bowel sounds are present. When she is examined vaginally, mucopus exudes from the cervical os. Movement of the cervix elicits pain in the lower abdomen, and she is tender in both vaginal fornices. A urine test for pregnancy is negative.

What Are the Most Likely Diagnoses?

The clinical findings strongly support the diagnosis of PID: bilateral abdominal tenderness, pain on moving the cervix, and tenderness in both vaginal fornices. An additional sign is that of inflammation of the endocervical canal. In the case of ectopic pregnancy, tenderness is usually unilateral and not bilateral as is usually found in PID. Clinical signs, however, are unreliable in differentiating between ectopic pregnancy and PID. In acute appendicitis tenderness in the right iliac fossa is more likely than bilateral tenderness as in this case.

Table 14.2 shows the organisms associated with PID. In geographical areas where the prevalence of gonorrhoea is low, such as the United Kingdom, *Chlamydia trachomatis*is the most common cause of PID.

As the diagnosis is likely to be PID, the GP refers Sarah to a Sexual Health clinic where the history and physical findings are confirmed. A serum level of human chorionic gonadotrophin (hCG) is <100 m I.U./mL. Gram-stained smears of urethral and

TABLE 14.2. Micro-organisms associated with pelvic inflammatory disease.

Chlamydia trachomatis
Neisseria gonorrhoeae
Mycoplasma genitalium
Anaerobic[a] and facultative bacteria, including: *Peptostreptococcus* spp.,
   Prevotella spp., *Gardnerella vaginalis*

[a]Particularly in older women, in those using an intrauterine contraceptive device, and in those with suppurative disease.

endocervical material are prepared as described in Case 2, and specimens are sent for the detection of gonococcal and chlamydial infections by nucleic acid amplification assays.

The Gram-stained smear of cervical exudate shows large numbers of polymorphonuclear leucocytes (>30 per ×1,000 microscopical field), but Gram-negative diplococci are not seen in this or in the urethral sample.

What Is Your Next Course of Action?

Although the low levels of hCG make pregnancy unlikely,[1] if there is any doubt, referral to a gynecologist is advised. Abdominal and/or transvaginal ultrasonography, together with knowledge of the hCG levels, can be useful in the diagnosis of ectopic pregnancy.

Although the finding of many white cells in the cervical specimen makes alternative diagnoses less likely, this test has a low positive predictive value. Having made a presumptive diagnosis of PID, however, Sarah should be treated before the results of the microbiological laboratory tests are available. There is some evidence that delay in initiating therapy is associated with increased subsequent morbidity, including the risk of infertility due to tubal

---

[1]Serum chorionic gonadotrophin (hCG) assays on serum and urine can detect pregnancy within 7–10 days and 14–18 days post-ovulation, respectively. It is therefore possible to diagnose pregnancy before the first missed period.

TABLE 14.3. Drug regimens for the treatment of mild to moderate pelvic inflammatory disease.

Ceftriaxone 250 mg as a single intramuscular injection
PLUS
Doxycycline 100 mg twice daily by mouth PLUS metronidazole
    400 mg twice daily by mouth, both given for 14 days
OR
Ofloxacin 400 mg twice daily by mouth PLUS metronidazole 400 mg
    twice daily by mouth both given for 14 days

---

fibrosis, increased risk of ectopic pregnancy from damage to ciliary motility, and chronic pelvic pain resulting from pelvic adhesions.

Table 14.3 shows the outpatient drug regimens used in the treatment of mild to moderate PID. In severe disease,[2] initial treatment is by the parenteral route, with a switch to oral therapy 24 h after clinical improvement.

Paracetamol is provided as analgesia, and Sarah is advised to abstain from sexual intercourse until she and her partner has completed treatment.

As women with mild PID are less likely to have anaerobic bacteria isolated from the uterine tubes than those with severe, suppurative infection, metronidazole may be discontinued if the patient is unable to tolerate his drug.

Partner notification is undertaken, and her partner attends the next day for treatment. He is symptomless, and a subsequent urine sample for the detection of C. trachomatis and N. gonorrhoeae yields negative results. Nevertheless, as false-negative results for chlamydiae can occur, he receives empirical treatment with a single oral dose of 1 g of azithromycin.

Sarah is reviewed 72 h after initiation of therapy with doxycycline and metronidazole. Her abdominal pain has improved

---

[2] Severe disease is associated with fever (temperature $>38°C$), malaise, anorexia, and vomiting. There is tenderness and guarding in the lower abdomen. The total white cell count in the peripheral blood is elevated and both the erythrocyte sedimentation rate (ESR) and the C-reactive protein concentration are raised, particularly in chlamydial PID.

considerably, and she is tolerating the antimicrobial regimen well.
Chlamydia trachomatis *but not* N. gonorrhoeae *was detected in the*
endocervical specimen taken at the first attendance.

It is recommended that patients with PID are reviewed 4 weeks
after therapy to ensure that the clinical response has been satisfactory and that partner notification has been completed (see Case 6).

Six months later, Sarah has now married her partner and both
wish to start a family. She has heard that chlamydia and PID may
cause infertility and wishes to discuss this with you.

In gonococcal and chlamydial salpingitis, the inflammatory process affects chiefly the mucosal lining of the uterine tubes, the
organisms having ascended from the endocervical canal by way
of the endometrium. There is destruction of tubal epithelium and
a purulent exudate fills the lumen. If untreated, fibrous adhesions
form within the tube and tubal infertility may result. However, the
magnitude of the risk of infertility is difficult to quantify. Scan-
dinavian studies conducted in the 1980s suggested that between
8 and 16% of women were involuntarily infertile after an episode
of PID. However, the spectrum of severity of PID varies widely,
and it is difficult to draw firm conclusions based on studies of
women who may have had more severe disease. (It is known
that among patients with only one episode of PID, the incidence
of tubal infertility is higher in those who have severe inflammation at laparoscopy than mild inflammation). Repeated or chronic
infection with *C. trachomatis* increases the likelihood of long-term
sequelae. In women with repeated episodes of pelvic inflammatory
disease, the risk of permanent tubal damage and consequent infertility doubles with each recurrent episode. This is not the case here,
however, as Sarah has experienced only one episode of mild-to-
moderately severe PID.

A recent study suggested that about 7% of women who had ever
been treated for chlamydial infection had infertility, a lower rate
than previously reported. This is therefore reassuring for Sarah and
her partner.

Case 15
A Young Woman with Genital Lumps

A 20-year-old woman, Linda, attends you as her General Practitioner. For the past 2 weeks she has noticed several swellings in the genital area. These are painless, but mildly itchy. She has not noticed lumps elsewhere on her body and she has not had generalized itch. Her general health is good, she is not receiving any medication, and she has no significant past medical history. Her periods are regular, the most recent having been 1 week previously. For the past 4 months she has been in a regular relationship with a 22-year-old man who has not noticed any genital abnormalities. Condoms are almost always used for vaginal intercourse. About 7 months ago she separated from her previous partner with whom she had been in relationship for 3 years. She has had no other sexual partners.

What Conditions Would You Consider in the Differential Diagnosis?

Table 15.1 indicates the most common causes of anogenital "lumps." Scabies would be an unlikely diagnosis as itch is not the principal feature in this case: it is mild, and localized to the genitalia. Lichen planus can be associated with itchy genital lesions, and usually, but by no means always, skin lesions are noted elsewhere. Condylomata lata may be the only feature of late secondary syphilis, but syphilis is uncommon in women in the UK.

The diagnosis is clinical. In this case, examination shows multiple cauliflower-shaped, fleshy, hyperplastic warts (condylomata acuminata) on the labia minora, at the introitus, and on the

A. McMillan, *Sexually Transmissible Infections in Clinical Practice*, 97
DOI 10.1007/978-1-84882-557-4_15,
© Springer-Verlag London Limited 2009

TABLE 15.1. Causes of anogenital lumps in women.

- Anogenital warts
- Molluscum contagiosum
- Normal anatomical features, such as pilosebaceous glands and vestibular papillae.
- Skin tags
- Scabies
- Seborrhoeic keratosis
- Lichen planus
- Condylomata lata (secondary syphilis)

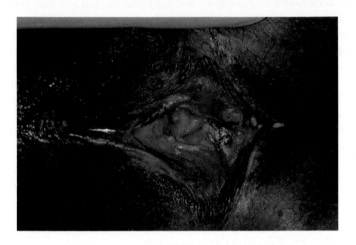

FIGURE 15.1. Warts on labia minora and perineum.

perineum (Fig. 15.1).[1] The vagina and uterine cervix appear normal.

---

[1] Other morphological types of warts occur on the genitalia:

- Papular warts, appear as flesh-colored papules.
- Keratotic warts that are crusted, resembling skin warts. They tend to be found in dry areas such as on the external labia majora or pubic skin.

Linda is very upset when she is given the diagnosis. She cannot understand why she but not her partner has warts.

What Information Do You Provide?

There is good epidemiological evidence that the virus causing the majority of anogenital warts – the human papillomavirus (HPV) types 6 and 11[2] – is acquired sexually. Uncommonly in adults, anogenital warts are caused by HPV types 1, 2, or 4, the types associated with common skin warts, and have most likely been acquired through auto-inoculation.

There is evidence that most HPV types 6 and 11 infections are transient and that the majority are symptomless or produce lesions that can only detected by detailed clinical examination, facilitated by magnification. As anogenital warts can have a long pre-patent period – a median of 3 months – it is usually impossible to tell when an individual has acquired his or her infection. The appearance of HPV lesions during a long-term relationship does not necessarily indicate infidelity.

How Would You Manage the Warts in This Case?

Anogenital warts are caused by a virus for which there is no antiviral treatment. Although most anogenital warts in immuno-competent patients eventually undergo spontaneous regression (cell-mediated immune responses are important in this process), treatment is offered to the majority of affected individuals with moist hyperplastic condylomata acuminata to reduce the risk of secondary infection and to alleviate anxiety. It must be explained

---

[2]On the basis of nucleic acid studies, more than 100 types have been reported. Four of the most common HPV types that infect the genital tract are HPV-6, HPV-11, HPV-16, and HPV-18. The former two types are found in hyperplastic anogenital warts, and, as they are not associated with cervical cancer, are designated "low-risk" types. Types 16 and 18, however, are frequently detected in anogenital cancers and are classified as "high-risk" types. Infection with multiple viral types, however, is common.

to the patient that treatment can be prolonged and that recurrence is common after the warts have been eradicated by treatment. She should be reassured, however, that the lesions will eventually regress permanently.

The exclusion, detection and, if required, treatment of other sexually transmitted infections in the affected individual and the sexual partner(s) are essential first steps (Cases 1 and 2). Before initiation of wart therapy, it is important to attend to any other local infection whether sexually transmitted or not. For example, in women, any cause of vaginitis or discharge must be discovered and eradicated, particularly trichomoniasis and candidiasis. Sometimes warts regress after local inflammation has been controlled.

Table 15.2 shows the most commonly used treatments for external anogenital warts.

TABLE 15.2. Treatments for anogenital warts.

Treatment	Comments
Podophyllotoxin	Antimitotic agent. Self-application. Useful for treatment of hyperplastic warts; less useful for keratinized lesions. Avoid in pregnancy
Imiquimod	Immunomodulatory agent. Self-application. Useful for hyperplastic warts; less useful for keratinized lesions. Safety in pregnancy not established, so avoid. Expensive
Cryotherapy	Ablative therapy. Useful for keratinized warts. Can be used in pregnancy. Clinic attendance necessary
Trichloroethanoic acid	Useful for small numbers of warts. Corrosive – care needs to be taken with its application. Not suitable for home use. Can be used in pregnancy
Electrosurgery	Useful for keratotic warts
Scissor excision	Useful for keratinized pedunculated warts, especially in perianal region. Local or general anesthesia needed
Laser	Useful for extensive warts (general anesthesia required). Not available in the majority of sexual health clinics

TABLE 15.3. Schedule for the first-line treatment of external genital warts.

Hyperplastic external genital warts, less than 10 in number or less than 5 cm² in area:
Cryotherapy with liquid nitrogen, repeated at two-weekly intervals for five cycles

OR

Podophyllotoxin 0.5% solution or cream (men) or 0.15% cream (women) applied twice daily for 3 consecutive days per week for up to 5 weeks

More extensive external genital warts:
Podophyllotoxin lotion or cream

OR

Imiquimod 5% cream, applied three times per week for up to 16 weeks.

Table 15.3 is a schedule for the treatment of external hyperplastic warts.

Linda opts for treatment with podophyllotoxin cream.

She should be instructed in the use of the cream, and preferably shown by the physician or nurse the method of application. It is also helpful to identify to her the warts that should be treated (normal anatomical structures can be mistaken for warts). Mild tenderness and burning are common, and Linda should be warned about this possible side effect.

She has considered changing from condoms to the combined oral contraceptive pill as contraception and wishes to know if it is necessary to continue condom use with her current partner. What is your advice?

It is reasonable to consider that he has already been infected with the virus – condom use has not been consistent. There are few data on which to inform your advice. However, there is some evidence that among men, the time to regression of penile warts is shorter among those who use condoms with their female partners than those who do not. This finding may be explained by the prevention of continued re-exposure to the virus. Condom use should therefore be encouraged.

She re-attends the clinic 5 weeks after initiation of therapy. The warts persist, but they have reduced significantly in number and size. Linda, however, is becoming impatient and requests an alternative treatment.

What Is Your Further Management?

If there is a partial response to initial therapy, a further cycle of the same can be used.

When there has been no response, however, a change to an alternative treatment is indicated: for example, cryotherapy to podophyllotoxin, or podophyllotoxin to imiquimod.

In this case, treatment is changed to imiquimod at the patient's request. What advice would you give?

The mode of action of imiquimod – stimulation of the immune system against the virus – is explained in simple terms, and it is stressed that an immediate effect on the warts may not be obvious (In one study, the median time to complete clearance of warts was 7 weeks).

A thin layer of imiquimod cream is applied to the wart area and allowed to remain on the skin for between 6 and 10 h (preferably overnight) before washing with soap and water. The cream is applied three times per week. If the patient develops marked pain or discomfort, it may be necessary to discontinue therapy. When symptoms have resolved, however, the drug can be re-introduced, although it may be helpful to reduce the frequency of application, for example, by instructing the individual to apply the cream once in the first week, twice in the second, and three times per week thereafter. Imiquimod cream may affect the latex condom, and Linda should be warned about this possibility.

Linda is prescribed a 4 week's supply of the cream and attends the clinic at the end of that time. She has had mild irritation around the warts, and some have regressed. She requests a further supply of cream.

As imiquimod may be used for up to a recommended maximum of 16 weeks, a further 1 month's supply is prescribed.

Linda has heard that warts can become cancerous and that she should have annual cervical cytological screening. How would you respond to this?

In the immunocompetent individual, malignant transformation of anogenital warts is rare. They are caused by HPV type 6 /11 which has a low potential risk for malignancy. Previously, annual cervical cytological examination was recommended in women with a history of anogenital warts. This is now known to be unnecessary, but she is advised to have smears at the nationally recommended time intervals. As there may be an increased risk of vulval and vaginal cancers in immunocompetent women who have had genital warts, the subsequent development of lumps should prompt medical review. In immunocompromised individuals, high-grade squamous intra-epithelial lesions (H-SILs) of the vulva, cervix, and anal canal are common and anogenital warts may become cancerous. More regular cytological cervical (and anal) screening is recommended in such individuals.

When she attends for review 1 month later, the warts have completely resolved, but although she is very much relieved, she would like to know the likelihood of recurrence. She also expresses concern about transmission of HPV to a future partner. She has separated from her partner, but has recently met a man with whom she wishes to start a relationship.

What Is Her Risk of Infecting Him, and Will Condom Use Prevent Transmission of HPV?

Warts may recur, but it is impossible to predict the likelihood of such an event. Recurrence is said to be more likely in those infected with multiple viral types, but testing for multiple infection is not routine. Interestingly, and consistent with its mode of action, the recurrence rate among individuals treated with imiquimod is lower than those treated by other methods.

Prevention of HPV infection is difficult. Genital warts are contagious, and, although lesions can be eradicated by treatment, there may be sub-clinical lesions from which HPV is shed either persistently or episodically. As judged by the detection of HPV DNA in cervico-vaginal samples, the median duration of viral shedding after infection is said to be 12 months. HPV DNA is no longer detectable in over 85% of women 18 months after infection. In the individual case, however, there is no means of ascertaining his or her infectivity.

There are conflicting data on the protective effect of condom use on HPV infection. The virus is transmitted by direct skin to skin or mucosal contact, and, as the virus is widespread in the anogenital region, it is unlikely that even consistent use of condoms will eliminate risk of infection. This theory has been substantiated in several studies. Other studies, however, have found that condom use protects against HPV acquisition, and there is now some evidence that the risk of acquisition of genital warts can be reduced.

Linda has heard that there is now a vaccine available for the prevention of HPV infection and asks for further information about this. What information is available about HPV vaccination, and who should be vaccinated?

Two vaccines are currently licensed for use: a bivalent vaccine (Cervarix®, GlaxoSmithKline) prepared from virus like particles (VLPs) of HPV 16 and 18, and a quadrivalent vaccine (Gardasil®, Merck) prepared from VLPs of HPV 6, 11, 16, and 18. For 5 years following vaccination, both vaccines show >90% efficacy in preventing persistent infection with the oncogenic types HPV 16 and 18, and the quadrivalent vaccine has about 99% efficacy in preventing infection with the HPV types associated with anogenital warts (types 6 and 11). In clinical trials, both vaccines have shown 100% efficacy in preventing cervical and vulval high-grade intraepithelial lesions (H-SILs). These are prophylactic vaccines, however, and no protective effect against H-SIL is seen in those women who have already been infected with oncogenic virus types.

A vaccination programme is being rolled out in many industrialized countries. In the United Kingdom, girls aged between 12 and 13 years are being offered vaccination with the bivalent vaccine, and there is a 3-year catch-up programme in which girls aged 13–18 years will be offered vaccine. As the bivalent vaccine will not prevent acquisition of HPV 6 or 11, the impact of the vaccination programme on the incidence of anogenital warts is unlikely to be significant. Males are not included in the programme, although H-SILs and anal cancer associated with the oncogenic types of HPV occur, particularly among men who have sex with men who are HIV-infected. There is also the possibility of infection being transmitted from a man to an unvaccinated woman.

Three doses of vaccine are given over a period of 6 months and studies have shown that high antibody levels can be achieved. The period of protection after primary vaccination, however, is uncertain, and it is still unclear as to whether or not booster does of vaccine will be required.

Case 16
A Young Woman with Genital Ulceration

Carol, a 23-year-old woman, attends you, her General Practitioner, with a 3 day history of pain and swelling of the vulva, slightly increased vaginal discharge, and pain on passing urine. When she examined herself using a mirror she noticed that there were many "cuts" all over the genital area. She has difficulty walking on account of the pain. Carol has been generally unwell for a few days and has felt feverish. She has not noticed a skin rash. Previously her general health has been good with no serious illnesses. She is not receiving any medication, and she has not applied ointments or lotions to her genitals. Her most recent menstrual period was 7 days previously and was normal. She has no previous history of genital ulceration. She has been in a regular relationship with Mark for 2 years, and she has had no other sexual contacts in that time. Mark, a 35-year-old man, attends with Carol. He has no symptoms and has no past history of sexually transmitted infections. Both he and Carol had had a sexual health screen shortly after they began their relationship. Neither was identified as having a sexually transmitted infection, although serological testing for previous exposure to herpes simplex virus was not undertaken (see Case 1). He tells you that his only sexual partner within the preceding 2 years has been Carol, but previously he has had several heterosexual relationships. They had vaginal and oral sex about 1 week previously. Condoms are used as contraception, but they have used the same brand for several months; they do not use lubricant.

A. McMillan, *Sexually Transmissible Infections in Clinical Practice*,   107
DOI 10.1007/978-1-84882-557-4_16,
© Springer-Verlag London Limited 2009

What Is the Most Likely Diagnosis?

The most likely diagnosis is primary genital herpes (see Table 16.1 for a classification of herpes simplex virus infection) – there is genital ulceration and systemic features (infrequent in non-primary or recurrent episodes).

Carol appears distressed and has difficulty sitting. The temperature is 37.6°C. The oral cavity and the pharynx appear normal. Multiple vesicles and ulcerated areas are found at the introitus, on the inner aspects of the labia minora, and on the labia majora (Fig. 16.1). The inguinal lymph nodes are enlarged and tender.

Do These Findings Confirm the Diagnosis of Primary Genital Herpes?

The clinical findings are consistent with a diagnosis of primary genital herpes. Table 16.2 shows other causes of anogenital ulceration. As the psychological impact of genital herpes is often considerable, however, it is good practice to confirm the diagnosis by laboratory testing. This is done by obtaining fluid from a vesicle or material from the base of an ulcer using a cotton wool-tipped

TABLE 16.1. Classification of herpes simplex virus infection.

1. *Primary infection.* This is an infection which may be asymptomatic, remain localized, or become generalized in an individual who has not been previously infected with either type of HSV as shown by a lack of antibodies to any herpes simplex virus
2. *Initial infection.* This denotes the first infection by one HSV type. It may be a *primary infection* in those *without* serological evidence of a previous herpetic infection (seronegative by a sensitive assay) or a *non-primary* in those *with* evidence of previous infection (seropositive). Clinically primary and non-primary initial infections may be indistinguishable on physical examination
3. *Latency.* There is apparent recovery but some virus remains dormant in nervous tissue, particularly in certain sensory ganglion cells; this is latency (latent means hidden)
4. *Recurrence.* The reactivated virus may on occasion initiate a peripheral lesion in the dermatome relating to the sensory ganglion. The lesion is referred to as a *recurrent lesion* and the phenomenon is *recurrence*

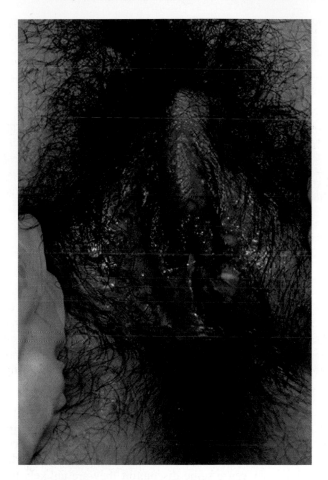

FIGURE 16.1. Vesicles and ulcers on vulva.

applicator stick and sending it in viral transport medium to the laboratory for the detection of specific HSV DNA using a nucleic acid amplification assay. The use of type-specific primers allows identification of the infecting HSV type. Alternatively, if a NAAT is unavailable, the specimen can be cultured in tissue culture; this, however, is a less sensitive diagnostic test.

In the case of herpes zoster, the lesions are confined to the dermatome, and not, as in Carol's case, widely distributed. Vulvo-vaginal candidiasis can produce vulval swelling and discomfort,

TABLE 16.2. Causes of anogenital ulceration.

Infective causes	Dermatological conditions	Systemic diseases
Varicella zoster virus infection	Trauma	Erythema multiforme
Treponema pallidum	Chemical burns	Pyoderma gangrenosum
Chlamydia trachomatis[a]	Lichen sclerosus et atrophicus	Behcet's syndrome
Haemophilus ducreyi	Lichen simplex	Crohn's disease
Klebsiella granulomatis	Erosive lichen planus	
Pyogenic ulceration	Pemphigus vulgaris	
Trichomonas vaginalis	Pemphigoid	
Candida spp.	Fixed drug eruption	
Sarcoptes scabiei	Other drug reactions (e.g., to Foscarnet)	
Mycobacterium tuberculosis[b]		
Entamoeba histolytica[b]	Squamous intraepithelial lesions of the vulva or penis Squamous cell carcinoma	

[a]Lymphogranuloma venereum genotypes.
[b]Rare

but pruritus is more likely than the severe pain reported in this case. The ulceration of primary syphilis is usually solitary and painless, but that of secondary syphilis may be multiple, although the lesions may cause some discomfort they are unlikely to produce severe pain. Chancroid (caused by *Haemophilus ducreyi*) is associated with multiple painful ulcers, but in Western Europe, it is usually diagnosed in individuals returning from geographical areas where the condition is prevalent, such as sub-Saharan Africa. The ulcer of lymphogranuloma venereum is usually solitary and symptomless, but multiple painful lesions may occur. As in the case of chancroid, most infections are recognized in individuals returning from tropical regions. The slow-growing, granulomatous ulceration of donovanosis, caused by *Klebsiella granulomatis*, is an unlikely diagnosis, most cases being identified in individuals from a few developing countries such as Papua New Guinea. Trichomoniasis can produce superficial vulval ulceration, but this is an unlikely cause of the painful lesions reported here. Scabies is associated with papular, often excoriated lesions on the genitalia; itch is the predominant symptom, and lesions would be found elsewhere on the body. Trauma or chemical burns can be discounted as causes of the genital ulceration in this case, and the lack of a history of drug ingestion rules out drug reactions. Lichen sclerosus et atrophicus can be associated with small eroded areas that may be sore. As Carol has an acute onset illness with systemic features, this is an unlikely diagnosis. Lichen simplex results from rubbing in response to itch and is often associated with fissuring. Carol's history is not compatible with this diagnosis. Lichen planus may also be associated with erosions at the introitus and inner aspects of the labia minora, but, again an acute onset with fever would be unusual. Pemphigus vulgaris can affect the vagina and vulva, and although associated with bullae, the blisters are easily ruptured producing erosions that are often painful. The history is not that of malignant disease, and the absence of associated features makes systemic diseases unlikely as a cause of Carol's genital ulceration.

What Is Your Immediate Management of Your Patient?

Antiviral drugs should not be withheld pending the results of the laboratory tests. The use of such agents within 5 days of the development of the clinical features of the infection has been shown to reduce the duration of the acute episode. The duration of new lesion formation, and the healing time are also shortened. Delay in initiating antiviral therapy beyond 5 days confers no benefit over placebo. Table 16.3 shows the antiviral drugs currently used in the management of primary or initial episode genital herpes.

Analgesia should be provided, and she should be advised to have frequent baths. When there is extensive ulceration of the inner aspects of the labia minora, the woman should be instructed to separate these during bathing to prevent the subsequent formation of fibrous adhesions.

TABLE 16.3. Drugs used for the treatment of primary or initial episode genital herpes.

Aciclovir 200 mg five times daily by mouth for 5 days

OR

Aciclovir 400 mg three times daily by mouth for 7–10 days

OR

Valaciclovir 500 mg twice daily by mouth for 5 days

OR

Famciclovir 250 mg three times daily by mouth for 5 days

When primary genital herpes arises during the course of a relationship, individuals consider that their partner has been unfaithful. It is therefore helpful at this stage to discuss a little of the nature of herpes simplex virus infection and to provide written information. In particular, it is important to point out that the majority of individuals (about 80%) infected with HSV, either type 1 (HSV-1) or type 2 (HSV-2), acquire the infection and never show features characteristic of either genital or orolabial herpes. Intermittent re-activation of virus in either the trigeminal or the sacral ganglia can result in centrifugal axonal transport[1] of infectious virions to skin or mucous membranes with the possibility of transmission to a partner. Exposure of a susceptible individual at this time through vaginal or anal intercourse, or oral–genital sex, can result in infection of that person with or without clinical features. As most episodes (about 90%) of sub-clinical shedding of virus last for only 2 days, it is quite by chance whether or not sexual contact occurs at the time of viral excretion. Mark has had previous sexual partners and it is possible that he acquired HSV through contact with one of these women. Alternatively, he could have acquired oral–labial HSV-1 when he was a child and transmitted reactivated virus during oral–genital sex.

---

[1]*Axonal transport.* The whole phenomenon requires translation of the virus from the periphery to the sensory ganglion and back again by way of, it is believed, the cytoplasm within the axon. The rate of translocation from the skin to the ganglion lies within the range of 2–10 mm per hour.

As individuals are often distressed at the first consultation, they are often not receptive to much information. For this reason it is useful to invite both Carol and Mark to re-attend about 1 week later for further counseling.

When you see Carol and Mark you have the results of the virological tests. Herpes simplex virus type 2 DNA has been detected in the material taken from the genital vesicles/ulcer. Her symptoms have improved markedly, but after accessing some internet sites, some of which she found alarming, she has a number of questions.

a) *Is there a cure for genital herpes?*
    No. Although the current antiviral drugs are useful in the treatment of primary or initial genital herpes, they do not prevent the development of latency in the dorsal root ganglia.
b) *What are the chances of the herpes recurring?*
    After the primary or initial infection there may be no further clinical manifestations throughout life. In the year following symptomatic primary genital herpes associated with HSV-2, however, *symptomatic* recurrence is common. It has been shown that up to 90% of individuals have recurrences, with a recurrence rate of about four to five episodes per year. (Significantly fewer recurrences are found in those who have had symptomatic primary HSV-1 genital infection: about one episode per year). In people who have had a prolonged initial illness (>35 days), the interval between primary infection and recurrence tends to be shorter and the recurrence rate to be twice as frequent as those with a less prolonged episode. Men tend to have more recurrences than women. In those patients who have had either HSV-1 or HSV-2 primary infections, the recurrence rates in the second year after the initial infection are significantly less than during the first year, although there is much variation in recurrence rates between individuals during that year. In many patients there is a reduction in recurrence rate in subsequent years, suggesting that the pool of reactivatable virus in the ganglia diminishes with time; the rate of decrease in recurrences, however, tends to become smaller with the passage of time. It should be noted, however, that about one-quarter of individuals have at least one more recurrence in year 5 than in year 1.

In recurrent genital herpes recurrences may be heralded by a prodromal sensation of tingling, occurring 30 min to 48 h before the appearance of lesions. In some patients, stabbing pains in the distribution of the sciatic nerve that last for several days may herald the recurrence. Several small vesicular lesions then appear and may coalesce. Lesions tend to increase in size over the first 3 days of the episode, remain static for about a week and resolve rapidly thereafter. The symptoms are substantially milder than those of the initial episode and constitutional symptoms are infrequent. Symptoms, however, tend to be more severe in women than in men.

The rate of *symptomless* shedding of HSV after recovery from an initial episode of genital herpes depends on the type of HSV. About 10% of women who have had primary HSV-1 infection and about 20% who have had primary or non-primary HSV-2 infection have symptomless excretion of virus at some time during the first year after the initial episode. Virus is more commonly excreted during the first 3 months than during subsequent months. About one-third of episodes of symptomless virus shedding occur in the 7 days preceding a symptomatic recurrence, and about one-fifth in the 7 days after such a recurrence. As has been noted with symptomatic recurrence (see above), sub-clinical shedding of virus is more likely to occur within 12 months of the initial episode of genital herpes than in subsequent years. Women who have frequent symptomatic recurrences (>12 per year) are also more likely to have sub-clinical shedding of HSV. There is no doubt that symptomless viral shedding is an important source of infection to sexual partners.

c) Am I at increased risk of cervical cancer?

No. Some years ago it was thought that HSV was associated with cervical caner. This has now been shown to be untrue.

For a discussion on the management of genital herpes in pregnancy, see Case 29.

Case 17
A Woman with Recurrent Genital Herpes

Carol (discussed in Case 16) attends you again some 2 years after the episode of primary genital herpes. She has become increasingly distressed by frequent recurrences of genital herpes – she has had about eight episodes in the past year. She understands that drugs are available for the treatment of recurrences but she is anxious to avoid taking medication unless it is considered necessary. Carol also is concerned that the virus could become resistant to the drugs should she use these regularly. She separated from Mark about 6 months previously, but she has recently met a man – William – with whom she would like to develop a relationship. Carol is most anxious that William who does not know that she has genital herpes does not become infected.

What Management Options Are Available for the Treatment of Recurrent Genital Herpes?

An approach to the management of the immunocompetent patient with recurrent genital herpes is shown in Fig. 17.1. Management, however, must be tailored to the needs of the individual and whose wishes must be taken into consideration.

I. *Supportive therapy.* Between patients, there is much variation in the frequency and severity of recurrences and hence the need for specific antiviral therapy is not uniform. In some patients, the recurrent episode is short-lived with few symptoms, and all that is required in management is careful attention to genital hygiene with saline bathing, and perhaps the topical application of an antiseptic agent such as povidone iodine 10% in an alcoholic solution. Other patients, however,

A. McMillan, *Sexually Transmissible Infections in Clinical Practice*, 115
DOI 10.1007/978-1-84882-557-4_17,
© Springer-Verlag London Limited 2009

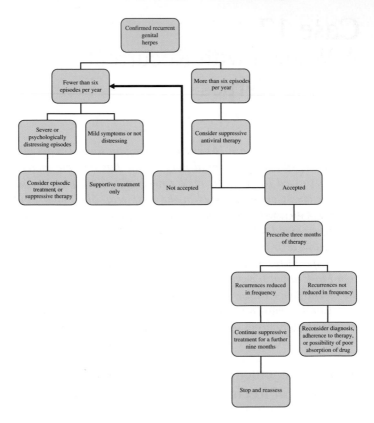

FIGURE 17.1. An approach to the patient with recurrent genital herpes.

have frequently recurring lesions and/or severe, prolonged symptoms, and in many individuals, including Carol, recurrent genital herpes is associated with psychological disturbance.

II. *Episodic antiviral therapy.* Although new lesion formation is usually inhibited when aciclovir is given by mouth to individuals with recurrent genital herpes, the effects on lesion progression are less pronounced than in initial disease, and so episodic treatment of patients with infrequent recurrences only confers marginal benefit. An exception would be if recurrences are severe or psychologically distressing. If episodic therapy is used, treatment should be initiated during the prodrome

TABLE 17.1. Drug regimens for the episodic treatment of recurrent genital herpes.

Aciclovir 800 mg three times per day for 2 days
OR
Valaciclovir 500 mg twice daily for 3 days
OR
Famciclovir 1000 mg twice daily for 1 day

(if there is one – see Case 16) or within 24 h of the appearance of symptoms. Patients should therefore be given a supply of drug to have ready for immediate use. Generally, shorter drug regimens than used for first-episode infection are effective (Table 17.1).

III. *Suppressive therapy.* Although individuals who have six or more recurrences per year are likely to show the most benefit in terms of reduction in frequency of recurrences, other people with fewer but severe recurrences, including those with neuralgia or other prodromal symptoms but who fail to develop genital lesions, may also benefit from suppressive therapy. In addition to the physical effects of suppressive therapy, there is a significant reduction in illness concern and anxiety. Table 17.2 shows the regimens recommended for suppressive therapy[1]. As there is a variable period of up to 1 year when recurrences are more frequent than in later months or years, it is better to postpone a decision about suppressive therapy until a pattern of recurrence can be established.

Carol decides that she will initiate suppressive treatment with aciclovir 400 mg twice daily. She is reassured to learn that there are few side effects – nausea, headache, and skin rash are unusual adverse events – and she is also relieved to learn that viral

---

[1] In Carol's case, the diagnosis of genital herpes had been confirmed virologically at her initial clinic attendance. However, if there had been no confirmation of the diagnosis, it is best to withhold suppressive treatment until this has been accomplished.

TABLE 17.2. Drug regimens used as suppressive therapy for frequently recurring genital herpes.

Aciclovir 400 mg twice daily by mouth

OR

Aciclovir 200 mg four times per day by mouth

OR

Valaciclovir 500 or 1000 mg once daily by mouth

OR

Valaciclovir 250 mg twice daily by mouth

OR

Famciclovir 250 mg twice daily by mouth

resistance to aciclovir is rare in the immunocompetent person. Aciclovir-resistant HSV is well recognized in the context of an immunocompromised infected individual.

Suppressive treatment for a short period of time is sometimes used in patients who wish to avoid recurrence at a particularly stressful time. For example, students who are studying for important examinations and have infrequent but distressing recurrences may benefit.

What Steps Can Be Taken to Prevent Transmission of Infection to William?

Unfortunately, vaccines for the prevention of acquisition of HSV are not available. There should be abstinence from sexual intercourse during symptomatic recurrence or during the prodrome, if any. As has been noted previously, transmission of infection can occur from individuals who are apparently symptomless. A sizeable proportion of people who have minor recurrent lesions can be taught to recognize these, and hence can avoid intercourse at that time. Consistent condom use by an infected male is considered to reduce the acquisition of HSV-2 by a female. There is no evidence that the risk of transmission from a female to a male is reduced; there is also no evidence that the use of the female condom reduces risk of transmission of the virus. Antiviral drugs reduce symptomatic and symptomless viral shedding, and it has been shown that during suppressive therapy with valaciclovir, the risk of transmission of HSV-2 to a sexual partner is reduced.

Carol consults you 3 months after initiation of suppressive therapy. She has had no recurrences, and she feels very much happier than previously. Her relationship with William continues, but condoms are used consistently for vaginal intercourse. William is still unaware that Carol has genital herpes.

You issue a prescription for a further 9 months supply of aciclovir. You also advise Carol that should she develop recurrence while taking the drug, she can increase the dose to 400 mg three times per day.

Disclosure to William should be discussed again. As noted above, consistent condom use and suppressive antiviral drugs can reduce but not negate the risk of transmission. In a developing long-term relationship it is perhaps better that disclosure occurs. The partner then enters a sexual relationship fully informed of the risks. Fears of allegations of infidelity are also allayed should he develop symptomatic HSV infection. A joint counseling session is often useful.

Carol re-attends you 9 months later. She has had no recurrences, and she tells you that William who is now aware of her infection has had no clinical features suggestive of genital herpes. Carol uses the combined oral contraceptive pill and condoms are not used during sexual intercourse.

What Advice Would You Give Now?

As there is some evidence that individuals who have received suppressive aciclovir for a year are less likely to have recurrent lesions after cessation of the drug than if they had not been treated, it is recommended that antiviral therapy should be discontinued at this time. It should be explained that it is not uncommon to have one or two recurrences within a few months of cessation of therapy, followed by long symptom-free periods. Therefore, a decision on re-initiating suppressive therapy should not be made until the individual has had at least two recurrences. (It is helpful to provide supply of an antiviral drug so that treatment can be initiated as soon as possible after the development of symptoms). Should more frequent recurrences develop, however, it is perfectly justifiable to offer further suppressive treatment. Suppressive aciclovir therapy has now been used for many years, and there do not appear to be long-term adverse events.

Case 18
A Gay Man with a Genital Ulcer

James is a 22-year-old man who attends you as a Sexual Health physician. He tells you that he had noticed a sore on his penis for about 5 days, and that this sore is increasing in size. You know that he has sex with men because he had asked you to undertake an HIV antibody test a year before for visa purposes, and he told you then that he was a sexually active gay man. You arranged for hepatitis A and B vaccination at that time, and a Health Adviser provided advice on risk reduction for the sexually transmitted infections.

What Further History Would You Wish to Elicit?

Specific enquiry should be made about the following:

- Is the "sore" painful or tender?
- Does it bleed easily?
- Has he had similar lesions in the past?
- Is there associated inguinal lymph node enlargement and if so, is uni- or bilateral, and are the enlarged glands painful or tender?
- Does he have lesions elsewhere on his body?
- What is his general health like?
- Has he taken any prescribed or illicit drugs within the preceding month, and if so when were these used?
- Has he had any sexually transmitted infections in the past?

The taking of a detailed sexual history is paramount (see Case 4).

James tells you that the sore is somewhat tender but does not bleed; he has had some discomfort in the right groin that he attributes to a groin strain sustained while playing football. He has not previously noticed any genital lesions. His general health

A. McMillan, *Sexually Transmissible Infections in Clinical Practice*, 121
DOI 10.1007/978-1-84882-557-4_18,
© Springer-Verlag London Limited 2009

is good, and he has not been aware of any sores elsewhere on his body or of skin rashes. He has not used any prescribed medication for at least 5 years, but over the past 3 years he has taken ecstasy about twice monthly when he has been clubbing. He has not been treated for any sexually transmitted infections in the past. He completed the course of hepatitis A and B vaccination and had been shown to have had a good antibody response.

James does not have a regular partner, but he has had sex with eight different men in the preceding 3 months. Most men he has met through the Internet, and he is able to contact three of them if necessary. All his recent partners have lived in the United Kingdom. His most recent sexual contact had been 1 week previously just before the sore developed. He tells you that he has both receptive and penetrative anal intercourse and that condoms are used consistently for anal sex. Although he performs and receives fellatio, he rarely uses condoms for oral sex.

What Do You Do Next?

You perform a detailed examination of the anogenital region. It is convenient to begin the examination by inspection of the lower abdomen for rash that may indicate early secondary syphilis (in about a third of patients, the primary lesion of syphilis is still present). Palpate the inguinal lymph nodes. In primary syphilis (chancre), there is usually bilateral inguinal lymph node enlargement; the glands are discrete, rubbery, and unless the chancre is secondarily infected, non-tender. In primary genital herpes, there is usually uni- or bilateral tender enlargement of the inguinal lymph nodes. Lymphogranuloma venereum (caused by the lymphogranuloma venereum genotypes of *Chlamydia trachomatis*) and chancroid (caused by *Haemophilus ducreyi*) are associated with tender and, usually, unilateral inguinal lymph gland enlargement and abscess formation.

The external genitalia are then inspected. During the examination, you should note the following:

* The anatomical site of the lesion or lesions.

- Whether the ulceration is single or multiple. For example, the lesions of genital herpes and chancroid are usually multiple, but primary syphilis generally presents as a single ulcer.
- Are the lesions tender, as may be found in genital herpes and chancroid?
- Is the lesion indurated, as is the case in *typical* primary syphilis? Note that this feature is often absent in extragenital chancres, such as in the anal canal.
- Does the lesion bleed easily? Chancroid is associated with multiple ulcers that bleed easily, whereas the primary lesion of syphilis tends not to bleed.

James has bilateral, non-tender inguinal lymph node enlargement. He has a single non-tender ulcer, measuring about 1 cm in diameter on the right side of the frenum (Fig. 18.1). It has a dull-red surface. When you palpate the lesion, you find that it is indurated[1] and that pressure produces serous exudate. There is no associated skin rash.

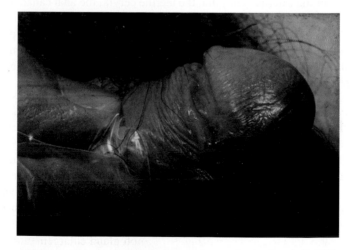

FIGURE 18.1. Solitary parafrenal ulcer.

---

[1]Indurated = hard; sometimes likened to cartilage or a button under the skin. Note that induration is not an invariable finding.

What Is the Most Likely Diagnosis?

The most likely diagnosis is primary syphilis. In recent years, there has been an increase in the incidence of early syphilis particularly among men who have sex with men, attending sexually transmitted infections clinics in the United Kingdom, continental Europe, Australia, and the United States. Although unprotected insertive and receptive anal intercourses are risk factors for acquisition of syphilis, in many cases the infection has been transmitted through unprotected oral–genital intercourse. Syphilis is caused by the spirochaete *Treponema pallidum* that is found in the fluid that exudes from the primary lesion or the moist mucosal or skin lesions of secondary syphilis (the dry skin lesions are not infectious). The organism invades the skin or mucous membrane where it initiates an inflammatory reaction in the dermis or submucosa that results in endarteritis with thrombosis and necrosis of the overlying epidermis or mucosal surface. Untreated, the primary lesion heals within 3–8 weeks. The primary lesion may be found on any part of the external genitalia, the uterine cervix, the anal canal, and the rectum. Lesions in the anal canal tend to be painful, tender, bleeding easily, and not indurated: thus in this anatomical site, primary syphilis resembles a traumatic anal fissure. Chancres may also occur on the lips, in the buccal cavity, tongue, tonsil, and pharynx.

How Would You Confirm the Diagnosis?

The diagnosis of primary syphilis can be made by dark field microscopy of the serum that exudes from the ulcer base. *T. pallidum* has a slender structure, with tight spirals and a characteristic motion.[2] Alternatively, *T. pallidum* can be detected by

---

[2]The published sensitivity of dark field microscopy varies between 79 and 97%. Both the sensitivity and specificity are dependent on the experience of the microscopist. Because of interference from commensal spirochaetes that are found in the normal flora of the genital and rectal mucosa, DGM is considered to be less reliable in examining rectal and non-penile genital

a polymerase chain reaction to detect specific DNA. Serological tests are used to confirm the diagnosis, but it should be borne in mind that in very early primary infection, the most commonly used screening tests – the treponemal enzyme immunoassay (EIA) or the Venereal Diseases Research Laboratory (VDRL) (or the Rapid Plasma Reagin test [RPR]) – may give negative results. It is therefore important to alert the laboratory that the patient may have primary syphilis so that more sensitive (but not routine) tests can be undertaken.

The serum from the ulcer on James' penis failed to show T. pallidum. *The serological results are as follows:*

Screening EIA test: NEGATIVE
VDRL test: NEGATIVE
Treponema pallidum particle agglutination test (TPPA): POSI-
TIVE (titer 1280)
Anti-treponemal IgM EIA: POSITIVE

These results confirm the clinical diagnosis.

What Is the Antimicrobial Agent of Choice, How Would You Administer It, and What Possible Reaction to Treatment Would You Warn Him of?

Table 18.1 shows the drug regimens used in the management of early infectious syphilis.

Penicillin is the treatment of choice. *T. pallidum* has not developed resistance to penicillin. The reason for prolonged treatment is that penicillin only acts on metabolically active organisms, and *T. pallidum* has a long generation time (30–33 h). James opts for benzathine penicillin.

---

lesions. DGM is not suitable for examining oral lesions because of the many commensal treponemes that occur in the mouth. DGM can be applied to the moist mucous lesions (condylomata lata or mucous patches) of secondary syphilis but as serological tests are virtually 100% sensitive at this stage there is little need for it.

TABLE 18.1. Drug regimens in the treatment of early syphilis.

Benzathine penicillin 2.4 MU in a single intramuscular dose, or repeated 7 days later

OR

Procaine penicillin G 600–750 mg once daily by intramuscular injection for 10 days

OR

Doxycycline[a] 100 mg twice daily by mouth for 14 days

OR

Erythromycin[a] 500 mg four times daily by mouth for 14 days

[a]May be used in patients with a history of penicillin hypersensitivity.

You have ascertained from the history that James is not hypersensitive to penicillin; nevertheless it is useful to invite him to remain in the clinic for about 30 min to ensure that there is no hypersensitivity reaction to the drug. James, however, may develop the Jarisch–Herxheimer Reaction (JHR); just over half of patients with primary infection develop this reaction. In primary syphilis the effects are usually mild. The reaction develops within 4 h of starting treatment, becomes most intense at 6–8 h, and resolves within 24 h.

The clinical phases are the following:

1. *Prodromal phase* with aches and pains.
2. *Rigor or chill.* Temperature rises by an average 1°C (range 0.2–2.7°C) 4–8 h after treatment.
3. *Flush.* Temperature reaches a peak, usually at about 8 h after the first injection and is associated with hypotension.
4. *Defervescence*, which lasts up to 12 h.

The JHR that occurs only with the first injection of penicillin is probably the result of cytokine activation following release of endotoxin from the injured treponemes.

What Else Would You Do?

In the control of syphilis, partner notification is paramount. Because of the long pre-patent period, sexual partners over the preceding 3 months should be notified. Because of the strong association between syphilis and HIV, it is worthwhile discussing HIV antibody testing. There is good epidemiological evidence that syphilis is associated with an increased risk of transmission or acquisition of HIV. This evidence is supported by the observation that the virus can be detected in the serum that exudes from the ulcerated lesions of primary or secondary syphilis.

James should also be offered testing for other STIs (see Case 4).

James should be followed up clinically and with serological testing 3, 6, and 12 months after treatment to ensure cure. The VDRL test is likely to remain negative, the anti-treponemal IgM EIA will become negative, the titer in the TPPA may decrease, but it is probable that the test will remain positive, possibly for many years.

What Is the Natural History of Untreated Early Syphilis?

Untreated, a proportion of patients develops benign tertiary syphilis (gumma formation), neurological (general paralysis of the insane, tabes dorsalis, or a combination of these conditions – taboparesis), or cardiovascular disease: about 15, 10, and 8% respectively.

The risk of neurosyphilis is increased some four-fold in HIV-infected patients, particularly when the CD4$^+$T-cell count is <350 per mL^3.

What Else Would You Do?

Case 19
An African Man with a Skin Rash

Charles, a 31-year-old post-graduate student from a country in sub-Saharan Africa, attends you, his General Practitioner, with a 6-week history of a slightly itchy skin rash all over his body. He has also noticed some swollen glands in his neck and under his arms. There are no other symptoms and he is not receiving any medication. The only significant illness in the past was malaria when he was a child. He returned to the United Kingdom 1 week ago after having spent 6 months in his native country. You refer him urgently to a dermatologist.

His temperature is 36.4°C. The dermatologist notes a generalized maculopapular scaling rash on the trunk (Fig. 19.1), arms, forearms, thighs, and upper legs. There are no palmar or plantar lesions. The pharynx is reddened but there is no ulceration. Significantly enlarged lymph nodes are palpated in the anterior and posterior triangles of the neck, the axillae, epitrochlear, and inguinal regions. The spleen is enlarged 1 cm below the costal margin but the liver is not enlarged. There are no other abnormal findings; in particular there are no anogenital lesions. Hematological indices and plasma enzyme tests of liver function are within normal limits.

A number of conditions enter the differential diagnosis of the skin rash (Table 19.1).

Lymphadenopathy in association with a skin rash may be found in pityriasis rosea, secondary syphilis, HIV infection, infectious mononucleosis, and rubella. The duration of the rash argues against the latter two infections, and the normal hematological indices make infectious mononucleosis an unlikely diagnosis.

As the diagnosis is uncertain, a skin biopsy is performed. There is an infiltration of lymphocytes and plasma cells in the superficial and deep dermis, particularly in relation to blood vessels and hair follicles (Fig. 19.2).

A. McMillan, *Sexually Transmissible Infections in Clinical Practice*, DOI 10.1007/978-1-84882-557-4_19, © Springer-Verlag London Limited 2009

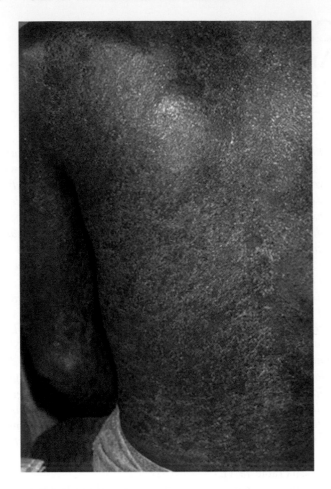

FIGURE 19.1. Maculopapular rash

The histology is not specific, but the dermatologist considers secondary syphilis as a possible cause and refers the patient to a Genitourinary Medicine physician.

The physician elicits a sexual history (see Case 1). He is married with two young children who live with their mother in Africa. She is 4 months pregnant. His most recent sexual contact with her had been about 1 month previously; he did not use condoms. Three

TABLE 19.1. Differential diagnosis of a maculopapular skin rash

Pityriasis rosea
Secondary syphilis
HIV infection
Infectious mononucleosis
Rubella
Psoriasis
Erythema multiforme
Lichen planus
Pityriasis lichenoides
Drug eruption

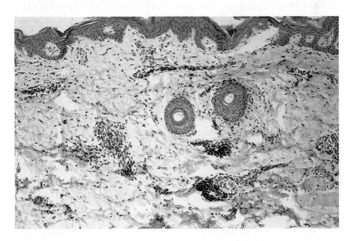

FIGURE 19.2. Lymphocytic and plasma cell infiltration of the superficial and deep dermis

months ago he had had unprotected sexual intercourse with a sex industry worker in a neighboring town. He has had no other sexual partners in the preceding 5 years. He does not recall ulceration of his penis.

With the history and physical findings, secondary syphilis, HIV, or both infections must be high on the list of differential diagnoses. Both conditions may be associated with skin rash and lymphadenopathy. Although the rash of secondary syphilis has been described as being non-itchy, this is not so in many cases. The long pre-patent period between possible exposure to infection and the development of the skin rash is unusual for primary HIV infection, but, of course, is consistent with that of secondary syphilis. Although fever may be a feature of both conditions, its absence does not preclude the diagnoses.

A rapid Venereal Diseases Research Laboratory (VDRL) test on undiluted serum is requested. The result is negative. Does this exclude the diagnosis of secondary syphilis?

No. One of the most serious disadvantages of the cardiolipin antigen tests, of which the VDRL is one, is the occurrence of the prozone phenomenon. This arises because agglutination is inhibited by excess antibody in the serum. The high protein concentration on the cardiolipin particles increases their charge, resulting in their mutual repulsion and preventing linking by antibody molecules. This is reversed by dilution of the serum and hence protein concentration.

The laboratory scientist repeated the VDRL test, using doubling dilutions of the patient's serum. She also undertook additional serological tests, the results being as shown in Table 19.2.

A fourth-generation HIV antigen/antibody test was negative, and tests for hepatitis B surface antigen and antibody against hepatitis B core antigen were negative. Tests for gonococcal and chlamydial infections (see Case 1) yielded negative results.

These test results confirm the clinical diagnosis of secondary syphilis and exclude HIV infection (the long interval between the presumed episode of risk and the duration of the clinical features preclude a false-negative HIV test). Charles is treated as described in Case 18.

TABLE 19.2. Results of serological tests for syphilis at initial attendance

- Screening anti-treponemal enzyme immunoassay (EIA): POSITIVE
- Venereal Disease Research Laboratory (VDRL) test: POSITIVE at a titer of 256
- *Treponema pallidum* particle agglutination (TPPA) test: POSITIVE at a titer of >5120
- Anti-treponemal IgM EIA: POSITIVE

Signs of secondary syphilis appear 7–10 weeks after infection or 6–8 weeks after the appearance of the primary lesion, if noticed.[1] Lesions of secondary syphilis result from the spread of *T. pallidum* throughout the tissues of the body and the immunological reactions of the host. Skin lesions are the most prominent feature of secondary syphilis, but other organs can be affected, including the liver (hepatitis) and the central nervous system (meningitis). Over a period of months the lesions of early syphilis (primary and secondary) heal and the disease becomes latent.

Charles is followed-up 3, 6, and 12 months after completion of treatment. Figure19.3 shows the changes in the serological tests over that time period.

Three months after completion of treatment, the anti-treponemal IgM EIA was positive, but this test became negative by 6 months.

As symptoms and signs of early syphilis regress spontaneously, cure of infection cannot be ascertained by resolution of clinical features. Serological tests for syphilis are therefore required to assess efficacy of treatment. Currently, non-treponemal tests such

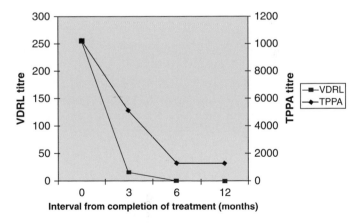

FIGURE 19.3. Changes in the VDRL and TPPA after completion of treatment

---

[1] Primary lesions of the uterine cervix, vagina or rectum may go unnoticed by the patient.

as the Venereal Diseases Research Laboratory (VDRL) or Rapid Plasma Reagin (RPR) tests are used for this purpose. After successful treatment of primary and secondary syphilis the VDRL titer declines four-fold at 3 months and eight-fold by 6 months. This is clearly shown in the present case. After successful treatment of early syphilis, anti-treponemal IgM declines rapidly and uniformly, and indeed was negative by 6 months is this case. Twelve months after treatment of secondary infection, however, the anti-treponemal IgM EIA is still positive in almost one-fifth of patients, even when the criteria for cure based on the non-treponemal tests (VDRL/RPR) are met. This test then does not appear to be satisfactory for determining cure of secondary syphilis.

Case 20
A Gay Man with Anal Discharge

A 20-year-old gay man, Eric, presents to a Sexual Health clinic with a 5-day history of constipation and discomfort in the anal region. He has noticed that his stools have been coated with "slime" tinged with blood. There are no other symptoms, his general health is good, and there is no relevant past history. His most recent sexual contact had been 1 week previously with an unknown British male with whom he had unprotected receptive anal intercourse. He has had no other sexual contacts within the preceding 6 months. Eric first became sexually active at the age of 17 years and he has had about 20 lifetime sexual partners. With the exception of his most recent sexual contact, insertive and receptive anal intercourse has been protected. He had a sexual health screen about 1 year previously when no infection was found. At that time he had been vaccinated against hepatitis A and B, and subsequent serological testing showed that he had a good antibody response to the latter vaccine. He has no known drug allergies.

What Is the Most Likely Cause of His Symptoms, and What Are Possible Causes?

The history is suggestive of a distal proctitis, Table 20.1 indicating the sexually transmissible causes of this.

Gonococcal or chlamydial proctitis is the most likely diagnoses in this case. Rectal gonorrhoea is symptomless in at least two-thirds of cases, and infection with the D – K genotypes of *Chlamydia trachomatis* is symptomless in about 90% of cases. Infection with the lymphogranuloma venereum (LGV) genotypes of *C. trachomatis*, however, usually causes a severe inflammatory

A. McMillan, *Sexually Transmissible Infections in Clinical Practice*,   135
DOI 10.1007/978-1-84882-557-4_20,
© Springer-Verlag London Limited 2009

TABLE 20.1. Sexually transmitted causes of a distal proctitis.
Neisseria gonorrhoeae
Chlamydia trachomatis:
• Genotypes D – K
• Genotypes L1, L2, L2a, and L3
Herpes simplex virus
Treponema pallidum

response, often with systemic features. Primary herpetic proctitis is often, but by no means always accompanied by perianal ulceration with considerable pain, low-grade fever, and sometimes urinary hesitancy from sacral nerve irritation. If the sexual history is accurate, primary syphilis of the rectum is unlikely, although proctitis can form part of the clinical picture of secondary infection even in the absence of skin lesions.

Eric looks well and he is not in distress. There is no abdominal tenderness or guarding, and neither liver nor spleen is palpable. The external genitalia appear normal and there is no significant inguinal lymph node enlargement. The perianal region is normal. During anoscopy, the normal vascular pattern of the distal rectal mucosa is absent,[1] and mucopus is noted in the lumen of the rectum. The mucosa appears normal beyond 12 cm from the anal margin.

The findings confirm a diagnosis of distal proctitis.

What Is Your Immediate Management?

Rectal specimens are taken for the identification of *Neisseria gonorrhoeae*, *C. trachomatis*, and herpes simplex virus, as described in Cases 4 and 16. In addition, a Gram-stained smear is prepared for immediate microscopical examination. If Gram-negative diplococci are identified in the smear, a *provisional* diagnosis of rectal

---

[1] Although absence of the normal vascular pattern of the mucosa is a feature of proctitis, visible vasculature is commonly absent in the distal 10 cm of the normal rectum.

gonorrhoea can be made and specific treatment initiated without delay. The sensitivity of the test on rectal specimens, however, is only between 70 and 80%, and, as other species of *Neisseria*, particularly *N. meningitidis*, which are morphologically identical to the gonococcus, are commonly found in the rectum, the specificity of this test may be low.

Microbiological tests for infections at other anatomical sites are also undertaken, and a blood sample is taken for serological testing for syphilis and HIV.

Gram-negative diplococci (see Case 7*) are identified within the cytoplasm of the numerous polymorphonuclear leucocytes noted in the rectal smear.*

The presumptive diagnosis is rectal gonorrhoea and treatment is given. The treatment regimens described in Case 7 are as efficacious in the treatment of rectal infection as they are in that of genital tract gonorrhoea. As at least one-quarter of men with rectal gonorrhoea have concurrent chlamydial infection, empirical treatment for this should be given simultaneously. Although data on its efficacy in treating chlamydiae in the rectum are scant, azithromycin in a single oral dose of 1 g is the most commonly used drug. Alternatively, doxycycline in an oral dose of 100 mg twice daily for 7 days may be given. Treated patients should be reviewed a week after completion of treatment for reasons discussed in Case 7.

Eric is treated with single oral doses of cefixime and azithromycin and is reviewed 1 week later. He is now symptomless, he has had no adverse events from treatment, and he has had no sexual contact in the intervening period. The laboratory tests confirmed the diagnosis of gonorrhoea and C. trachomatis *DNA was detected in a rectal specimen. Genotyping showed that the DNA detected was not of the LGV genotype. Other tests, including those for syphilis and HIV were negative. He has been unable to identify and contact the man who was the source of his infection.*

Rectal gonorrhoea is an important infection to identify. As stated above, it is often symptomless, but may be complicated by perianal abscess formation, and, rarely, disseminated infection (see Case 24). In addition, it is clear that gonorrhoea facilitates the transmission of HIV infection.

Counseling on risk reduction for the acquisition of sexually transmitted infections, including HIV, should be undertaken routinely. In this case, serological tests for syphilis should be repeated 3 months after the sexual risk, the pre-patent period of syphilis being between 10 and 90 days. Similarly, repeat HIV testing is also indicated at that time, or earlier if indicated.[2]

---

[2]Earlier testing may be indicated if the person is a known contact of an HIV-infected individual, or if he/she develops clinical features suggestive of primary HIV infection.

Case 21
A Gay Man with a Rash, Lymphadenopathy, and Fever

Thomas, a 20-year-old gay man, presents to a Sexual Health clinic 2 days after developing fever and a skin rash. He has felt generally unwell for about 5 days, and he has had a sore throat, mouth ulcers, headache, and generalized aching in his muscles and joints. He has also noticed swollen glands in his neck. Until now his health has been good, he has had no significant previous illnesses, and he is not receiving prescribed drugs. Thomas does not know to which infections he has been immunized. He is concerned that he might have acquired syphilis because a friend had told him that one of his sexual partners had been treated for this infection about 2 months previously. Thomas thinks that he had only unprotected oral–genital sex with this man about 3 months ago. He has been sexually active for about 3 years and he has had about 25 different sexual partners in that time. In the preceding 3 months he has had sexual contact with five different men. Although he is aware of safer sexual practices, he occasionally has unprotected anal intercourse, particularly when he has consumed considerable quantities of alcohol. Ten days prior to his clinic attendance, he had unprotected receptive anal intercourse with an unknown man whom he had met at a sex club. He regularly uses inhalational nitrites (poppers) during sex, and he occasionally uses "ecstasy."

What Conditions Might Cause These Symptoms?

Sexually transmissible causes of fever, skin rash, and lymphadenopathy are shown in Table 21.1.

Secondary syphilis must be high on the list of differential diagnosis, as he has had sexual contact with a male possibly infected with syphilis. The pre-patent period would be in keeping with a

A. McMillan, *Sexually Transmissible Infections in Clinical Practice*, 139
DOI 10.1007/978-1-84882-557-4_21,
© Springer-Verlag London Limited 2009

TABLE 21.1. Sexually transmissible causes of fever, skin rash, and lymphadenopathy.

Secondary syphilis
Primary HIV infection
Infectious mononucleosis
Hepatitis B
Cytomegalovirus
Herpes simplex virus

diagnosis of secondary syphilis, and, although Thomas apparently did not have unprotected anal intercourse, oral–genital sex is a well-recognized means of acquisition of *Treponema pallidum*. The clinical features and diagnosis of secondary syphilis are described further in Case 19.

Unprotected receptive anal intercourse is a high-risk factor for the acquisition of HIV, and this infection must also feature prominently on the list of differential diagnoses. Clinical features of acute HIV infection develop in between 50 and 70% of individuals, the pre-patent period varying from 1 to 6 weeks. In symptomatic patients, there is a rapid onset of fever, malaise, headache, myalgia, sore throat, and swollen lymph glands. Diarrhea may also be a feature, and some patients develop oral, genital, or anal ulceration. A symmetrically distributed non-pruritic macular or maculopapular skin rash may be found on the trunk and limbs, and some affected people show signs of immunodeficiency, for example, oral candidiasis. Neurological features include meningitis, acute encephalitis, and peripheral neuropathy.

In a young patient, infectious mononucleosis, caused by Epstein–Barr virus, can cause the symptoms described here. An erythematous macular or maculopapular rash is a feature in a few patients, but oral ulceration is uncommon.

Acute hepatitis B infection can be associated with fever, lymphadenopathy, and an urticarial skin rash.

In acute cytomegalovirus infection, pharyngitis and prominent lymphadenopathy are less commonly found than in infectious mononucleosis.

Primary herpetic gingivostomatitis can be associated with fever, lymphadenopathy, and erythema multiforme.

Other causes of a glandular fever-like illness include rubella, drug reactions, for example, to phenytoin, streptococcal pharyngitis with erythema multiforme, and acute toxoplasmosis (a skin rash is an unusual feature).

Thomas appears listless. His temperature is 37.8°C, and his pulse rate is 90 per minute. There is a maculopapular rash on the trunk and arms (Fig. 21.1) and three aphthous-like ulcers are noted on the gingival margin; the pharynx is markedly reddened,

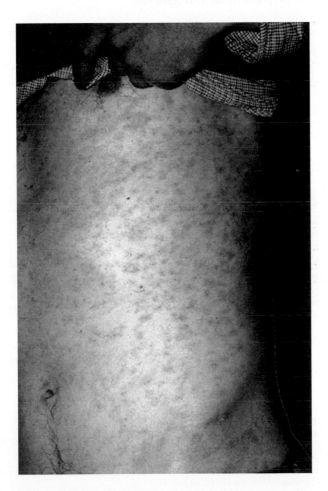

FIGURE 21.1. Maculopapular rash on trunk.

but exudate is not seen. There is significant but minimally tender enlargement of the anterior and posterior cervical lymph glands. Neither the liver nor the spleen is palpable. There are no clinical signs of meningitis, and a brief neurological examination shows no abnormalities.

Has the Physical Examination Help in the Differential Diagnosis?

In the absence of tender enlargement of the liver, viral hepatitis is unlikely, and the finding of pharyngitis with significant lymphadenopathy is unusual in acute cytomegalovirus infection.

Oral ulceration can be a feature of secondary syphilis and of primary HIV infection.

The results of hematological and biochemical tests undertaken at Thomas's initial clinic attendance are shown in Table 21.2.

TABLE 21.2. Results of hematological and biochemical tests.

Hematology:

Hemoglobin	146 g/L (130–180 g/L)[a]
Total leucocyte count	3.9×10^9/L $(4.0–11.0 \times 10^9$/L)
Neutrophils	2.9×10^9/L $(2.0–7.5 \times 10^9$/L)
Lymphocytes	0.8×10^9/L $(1.5–4.0 \times 10^9$/L)
Monocytes	0.2×10^9/L $(0.2–0.8 \times 10^9$/L)
Basophils	0.04×10^9/L $(0.05–0.1 \times 10^9$/L)
Eosinophils	0.17×10^9/L $(0.04–0.4 \times 10^9$/L)
Platelets	94×10^9/L $(150–350 \times 10^9$/L)
Blood film	Normocytic, normochromic erythrocytes. Platelets appear reduced in numbers. No atypical lymphocytes seen.
Monospot test	Negative

Biochemical tests on serum:

Bilirubin	12 μmol/L (2–17 μmol)
Alanine aminotransferase (ALT)	62 U/L (10–50 U/L)
Alkaline phosphatase	116 U/L (40–125 U/L)
Gamma glutamyl transferase	42 U/L (5–55 U/L)
Albumin	44 g/L (35–50 g/L)

[a]Normal values are shown in parentheses.

How Would You Interpret These Laboratory Findings?

Lymphopenia and thrombocytopenia, with a minimally elevated serum alanine aminotransferase level are the salient laboratory abnormalities. This is not the hematological picture seen in infectious mononucleosis: there is a lymphocytosis (up to 15×10^9/L), and the majority of cells in the peripheral blood have an atypical morphology. In addition, the Monospot test, a rapid screening test for heterophil antibodies, is positive in more than 85% of cases. In secondary syphilis, the peripheral blood leucocyte count is often normal, although a lymphocytosis may be found.

Leucopenia and lymphopenia, sometimes with the appearance of atypical lymphocytes in the peripheral blood, may be found in acute viral hepatitis. The alanine aminotransferase level, however, would be considerably higher than that found in this case.

The laboratory findings in this case would be consistent with a diagnosis of primary HIV infection. Lymphopenia, thrombocytopenia, and mildly elevated hepatic transaminase are often found in the first week after HIV infection. During the second week, there is a lymphocytosis, secondary to an increase in the number of CD8$^+$ T-cells, and abnormal lymphocytes (CD8$^+$ T-cells) are be found in the peripheral blood. The proportion of abnormal cells, however, is lower than that found in infectious mononucleosis or in acute cytomegalovirus infection.

A sample of serum is tested for HIV using a fourth-generation test that is designed to detect IgG and IgM antibodies and HIV p24 antigen. Serological tests for syphilis (an enzyme immunoassay [see Case 18]), hepatitis B (hepatitis B surface antigen and antibody against hepatitis B core antigen – see Case 32), rubella, Epstein–Barr virus, cytomegalovirus, and Toxoplasma gondii *are undertaken. Thomas is also screened for other sexually transmitted infections as described in Case 4.*

The test for HIV is positive, but serology for the other viral infections, syphilis and for T. gondii *shows no evidence of recent infection.* Neisseria gonorrhoeae *is cultured from the rectum, and* Chlamydia trachomatis *DNA is detected by a nucleic acid amplification assay performed on rectal material.*

The fourth-generation tests for HIV that detect antibody and antigen are much more sensitive than previous test systems for the identification of acute HIV infection, and the window period between infection and a positive test result has been considerably reduced. False-negative results may occur, however, and if there is strong clinical suspicion that a patient has acute infection, the test should be repeated and the plasma tested for HIV RNA. A positive result should always be confirmed by submitting a second serum sample (technical errors can occur, for example, through mislabeling of blood tubes). Most laboratories confirm a positive enzyme immunoassay result by immunoblotting (Western blotting).

Although serological tests can be negative in early primary syphilis, a negative result excludes secondary infection.

Unprotected receptive anal intercourse, particularly with ejaculation, is a high risk activity for the acquisition of HIV, and concurrent infection with gonorrhea and chlamydial infection increase that risk significantly. There is no doubt that the prevalence of sexual risk-taking has increased in recent years among men who have sex with men (MSM), as evidenced by the continued transmission of HIV and the increased prevalence of other STIs such as syphilis and gonorrhea among MSM in many industrialized countries. Although risk-taking is often attributed to excess use of alcohol, data from numerous studies have failed to find such an association. The use of inhalational nitrites, however, has been associated with unsafe sexual practices.

The confirmatory tests for HIV are positive. The plasma RNA viral load is $>1 \times 10^6$ per mm^3. A genotypic resistance assay shows no evidence of viral resistance to any class of antiretroviral agents.

The diagnosis is made. At this stage it is good practice to determine if drug-resistant virus has been acquired. This knowledge will facilitate the future choice of antiretroviral therapy when this is indicated.

Currently the treatment of acute HIV with antiretroviral agents is controversial, and neither this aspect of his management nor his subsequent follow-up will be discussed here.

Section B

Case 22
A Young Man with Persistent Urethral Symptoms

Pierre, a 23-year-old student, attends a Sexual Health clinic with a 5-day history of urethral discharge and mild pain on micturition. There are no other urological symptoms. He had been treated 1 month previously for non-gonococcal urethritis (NGU) with a single oral dose of 1 g of azithromycin. Within several days of that treatment, he became symptom free. He tolerated the medication well without vomiting or diarrhea. He has been in a regular sexual relationship for 3 months with a 19-year-old woman who attended the same clinic and was screened for sexually transmissible infections. As is routine clinic practice she was treated with azithromycin at that time. Neither Chlamydia trachomatis *nor* Neisseria gonorrhoeae *was detected in either partner, and* Trichomonas vaginalis *was not identified in a saline-mount preparation of vaginal material. They abstained from sex for 1 week after treatment, but since then they have had regular unprotected vaginal intercourse. Neither partner has had sexual contact with another person for at least 4 months.*

How Would You Account for the Recurrence of His Presumed Urethritis?

Recurrent or persistent urethritis, occurring within 30–90 days of treatment of NGU occurs in up to 20% of cases. The etiology of recurrent urethritis is often uncertain, but unprotected intercourse with an untreated partner is a possible cause. If the history is accurate, this is unlikely in this case. *Mycoplasma genitalium* has been implicated as a cause in up to 20% of cases of NGU. Significant failure rates have been reported after treatment of *M. genitalium*

A. McMillan, *Sexually Transmissible Infections in Clinical Practice*, 147
DOI 10.1007/978-1-84882-557-4_22,
© Springer-Verlag London Limited 2009

NGU with a 1 g single oral dose of azithromycin. The absence of *T. vaginalis* on direct microscopy vaginal material from his partner does not exclude this organism as the cause of recurrent NGU (see Case 10).

A mucoid urethral discharge is noted, and a Gram-stained smear shows >30 polymorphonuclear leucocytes per ×1,000 microscopical field but Gram-negative diplococci are not identified. Trichomonas vaginalis *is not detected in a saline-mount preparation of urethral discharge. Urinalysis does not detect blood, protein, or nitrites. A first-voided specimen of urine is obtained for the detection of C.* trachomatis, *and a mid-stream specimen is sent to the laboratory for culture for urinary tract pathogens. Nucleic acid amplification methods for the detection of* M. genitalium *and* T. vaginalis *are unavailable.*

The findings confirm a diagnosis of non-gonococcal urethritis. In the absence of additional clinical features such as frequency, nocturia, and urgency, a urinary tract infection is an unlikely cause of his urethritis.

How Would You Manage This Case?

Table 22.1 shows recommended treatment regimens for recurrent of persistent urethritis.

TABLE 22.1. Recommended treatment regimens for recurrent or persistent non-gonococcal urethritis.

Azithromycin 500 mg as a single oral dose followed by 250 mg once daily for 4 days

OR

Erythromycin 500 mg four times per day for 21 days

PLUS

Metronidazole 400 mg twice daily for 5–7 days

Metronidazole should be included in the regimen because *T. vaginalis* has not been excluded as a cause of his urethritis.

As mentioned above, single-dose treatment with azithromycin often fails to eradicate *M. genitalium*. Good results, however, have been obtained with azithromycin given as a single oral dose of 500 mg followed by 250 mg once daily for 4 days. Some physicians are concerned about the development of resistance of *M. genitalium* to the macrolides, particularly following treatment with a single dose of azithromycin (*M. genitalium* is slow-growing and may therefore be exposed to sub-optimal concentrations of the drug). Treatment failure with doxycycline is well documented, and in vitro studies have shown that the sensitivity of *M. genitalium* to levofloxacin and ciprofloxacin is reduced. Moxifloxacin, however, given in an oral dosage of 400 mg once daily for 10 days has proved to be effective.

As his partner has been treated previously, further treatment of her is not indicated.

Pierre who was treated with the short course of azithromycin and metronidazole returns to the clinic 2 weeks later. Once again, C. trachomatis *was not detected at the above clinic attendance, and significant bacteriuria was not found in the mid-stream urine specimen. He still complains of urethral discharge and mild dysuria; there are no other symptoms. He had no adverse reactions to the medication. Examination confirms a mucoid urethral discharge with significant numbers (>5 per ×1000 field) of polymorphonuclear leucocytes in a Gram-stained smear.*

What Would You Do Next?

After treatment of urethritis, the inflammatory response in the urethra may take several weeks to resolve, even when the causative organism, if one was identified, has been eradicated. It is therefore worth reassuring him that the urethritis is likely to resolve spontaneously and that further antimicrobial treatment is not indicated.

He returns to the clinic 1 month later. His symptoms have not improved.

What Do You Do Next?

As an underlying urological abnormality may, rarely, cause recurrent or persistent urethritis, referral to a urologist is the next course of action. If no abnormalities are found, he should be strongly reassured about this is a benign condition that in most cases, will eventually resolve without sequelae. For example, there is no evidence that fertility is impaired.

Case 23
A Man with Severe Dysuria

A 21-year-old man, James, attends a Sexual Health clinic with a 4-day history of severe pain on urination, associated with general malaise and feverishness. He does not have frequency of micturition, urgency, hesitancy, frank hematuria, or abdominal pain. He had unprotected receptive oral sex with a young woman whom he had met at a party 7 days previously; he did not have genital–genital contact with her. Before that encounter, his most recent sexual contact had been some 6 months previously with an ex-girlfriend.

He looks well. His temperature is 37.5°C. There is no skin rash and no conjunctivitis. There is marked meatitis (Fig. 23.1) and a mucoid urethral discharge. Genital ulceration is not noted. Several lymph nodes in the left inguinal region are enlarged and tender. Dipstick analysis shows no proteinuria, hematuria, or glycosuria.

Microscopy of a Gram-stained urethral smear shows about 5 polymorphonuclear leucocytes per ×1,000 field; Gram-negative diplococci are not identified.

What Two Sexually Transmissible Infections Would You Consider as the Most Likely Cause of His Urethritis?

The severity of the dysuria with the finding of urethral meatitis and inguinal lymphadenopathy suggests the possibility of either herpes simplex virus (HSV) infection or adenovirus infection. Both

A. McMillan, *Sexually Transmissible Infections in Clinical Practice*,   151
DOI 10.1007/978-1-84882-557-4_23,
© Springer-Verlag London Limited 2009

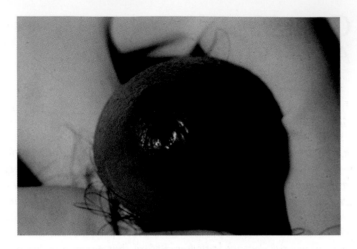

FIGURE 23.1. Meatitis.

primary HSV infection[1] and adenovirus infection may be associated with systemic symptoms as in this case. As the pre-patent period for both infections is short – between 4 and 10 days – consideration of this does not help in the differential diagnosis. The absence of external genital ulceration does not exclude urethral HSV infection that could have been acquired through oral–genital sexual contact. (In industrialized countries, almost half of all cases of primary genital herpes in young adults are caused by HSV type 1). Adenovirus infection can cause upper respiratory disease, and sometimes conjunctivitis. Urethral infection may result from insertive oral–genital contact with an individual who is excreting virus from the upper respiratory tract. (It is known that viral shedding can occur for a prolonged period after the initial infection). Although there have been several case reports of adenovirus-associated urethritis with conjunctivitis, the absence of the latter feature in this case does not exclude the diagnosis.

---

[1] This is an infection in an individual who has not been previously infected with either HSV type 1 or HSV type 2.

The severity of the dysuria with minimal signs argues against a diagnosis of urethral gonorrhea, a conclusion supported by the absence of Gram-negative diplococci in the Gram-stained smear.

Urethral infection with the oculogenital genotypes of *Chlamydia trachomatis* is unlikely to be associated with such severe dysuria. In any case, *C. trachomatis* is found uncommonly in the oropharynx, and the risk of transmission to the urethra during fellatio is considered to be small. Although there have been outbreaks of anorectal infection with the lymphogranuloma venereum genotypes of *C. trachomatis* amongst men who have sex with men, urethral infection appears to be rare, and the sexual history makes this a most unlikely diagnosis in this case.

How Would You Manage This Case?

Urethral material should be obtained from the urethra for the detection of HSV and adenovirus DNA by nucleic acid amplification methods. Although Gram-negative diplococci were not identified in smear microscopy, culture or a NAAT for *Neisseria gonorrhoeae* should be performed. A first-voided specimen of urine should also be obtained for the detection of *C. trachomatis* DNA.

Adenovirus infection is self-limiting and antiviral agents are not available for use in urethral infection. As the differential diagnosis includes HSV infection, he should be given a 5-day course of aciclovir, valaciclovir, or famciclovir (see Case 16). Many physicians would also give either a single oral dose of azithromycin or a 7-day course of doxycycline.

He returns to the clinic 7 days later. His symptoms have resolved, and the urethral meatus appears normal. HSV-1 was detected in the swab taken from the urethra, but the laboratory tests for adenovirus, N. gonorrhoeae, *and* C. trachomatis *were negative. He was counseled about genital herpes as described in* Cases 16 and 17.

Case 24
A Young Man with a Painful Swollen Knee Joint

A 23-year-old man, William, who works as a waiter, presents to his General Practitioner with a 6-day history of having a painful swollen right knee joint. For the past 3 weeks he has also noticed some stinging when passing urine. His GP suspects that he may have acquired a sexually transmitted infection and refers him to a Sexual Health clinic.

His GP has considered that the man may have urethritis, complicated by arthritis.

What Sexually Transmissible Infections May Be Associated with Arthritis?

Sexually transmissible infections associated with arthropathy include those shown in Table 24.1.

William attends the clinic 4 days later. He has now noticed pain and swelling of the left ankle joint, and he has developed a non-itchy, non-tender rash on his penis. He has also noticed that his eyes have become irritable. He has not had any recent episodes of diarrhea. There is no relevant past history, in particular he has had no previous joint or intestinal disorders, and he does not suffer from recurrent mouth ulcers. Although he plays football, he does not recall any recent significant injury. He lives in a large city in the United Kingdom and has not traveled into the countryside for more than 2 years. There is no family history of joint disease or of psoriasis. His only current medication is ibuprofen that was prescribed by his GP to control the joint pain. About 2 weeks before the onset of his urethral symptoms, he had unprotected vaginal intercourse with an unknown woman whom he had met at a party.

A. McMillan, *Sexually Transmissible Infections in Clinical Practice*, 155
DOI 10.1007/978-1-84882-557-4_24,
© Springer-Verlag London Limited 2009

TABLE 24.1. Sexually transmissible infections associated with arthropathy.

Chlamydia trachomatis
Neisseria gonorrhoeae
Treponema pallidum (secondary syphilis)
Mycoplasma genitalium
Ureaplasma urealyticum
HIV
Hepatitis B virus
Epstein–Barr virus
Shigella spp.
Campylobacter spp.

His temperature is 37.2°C, and his pulse 76 per minute. William has difficulty walking on account of pain in his right knee and left ankle joints, both of which are swollen and tender; the overlying skin is reddened. The left Achilles tendon is tender at its insertion into the calcaneum. Moist, glistening, red, sharply-defined macules with a polycyclic margin are found on the glans penis (circinate balanitis) (Fig. 24.1). Skin lesions elsewhere are not noted, and there are no oral lesions. The conjunctivae are reddened. There is a mucoid urethral discharge.

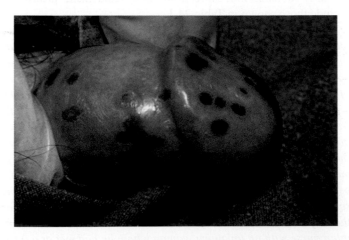

FIGURE 24.1. Circinate balanitis.

What Diagnoses Would You Consider?

The clinical features strongly suggest a diagnosis of reactive arthritis, the salient features of which are shown in Table 24.2. Reactive arthritis is one of the spondyloarthropathies that include ankylosing spondylitis, psoriatic arthritis, and the arthritis associated with inflammatory bowel disease and shares clinical features with these conditions. There is a strong association between these diseases and the major histocompatibility complex class I antigen HLA-B27: for example, the prevalence of HLA-B27 in patients with ankylosing spondylitis and reactive arthritis is between 85–95% and 30–80%, respectively.

Reactive arthritis may follow genital tract infection, particularly with *Chlamydia trachomatis*, and, less frequently *N. gonorrhoeae*, *Ureaplasma urealyticum*, and *Mycoplasma genitalium*, and is often referred to as sexually acquired reactive arthritis (SARA). Sexually acquired reactive arthritis is a disorder of young adults, the age of onset usually being between 18 and 50 years. Males are affected some 50 times more frequently than females. Intestinal

TABLE 24.2. Features of reactive arthritis.

Arthritis:
- Asymmetrical oligoarthritis affecting principally the joints of the lower limbs
- Monoarthritis
- Sacroiliac joint involvement
- Enthesitis (inflammation of ligamentous and tendinous insertions)
- Dactylitis (inflammatory involvement of a whole digit with tendovaginitis and arthritis

Extra-articular features:
- Ocular features:
  - Conjunctivitis
  - Anterior uveitis
- Skin and mucosal lesions:
  - Patchy loss of filiform papillae of the tongue
  - Psoriatic lesions (circinate balanitis and keratoderma blennorrhagica [pustular psoriasis])
  - Nail dystrophy
- Aortitis and cardiac conduction defects

infections, particularly with *Campylobacter* spp., *Shigella flexneri*, *Salmonella* spp., and *Yersinia enterocolitica*, can also trigger reactive arthritis.

The pre-patent period is variable, but the disease usually manifests itself 10–30 days after sexual intercourse or after an attack of dysentery or a dysentery-like illness. The mode of onset is variable, but commonly urethritis precedes the appearance of conjunctivitis, which is followed by arthritis. Any of the three features, however, may appear initially.

In this case there is oligoarthritis, enthesitis (inflammation of the insertion of the Achilles tendon), conjunctivitis, and circinate balanitis. Not all extra-articular manifestations of reactive arthritis need to be present to make the diagnosis. Other conditions, however, must be considered in the differential diagnosis (Table 24.3) and excluded by consideration of the clinical features and laboratory tests.

Gonococcal arthritis is the disease with which SARA is most often confused. Both conditions have urethritis and arthritis in common. Patients with disseminated gonococcal infection (DGI) often present with fever, migratory arthralgia, tenosynovitis, and skin lesions (painful, asymmetrically distributed hemorrhagic, or vesiculopustular lesions on an erythematous base [Fig. 24.2] that should not be confused with the psoriatic lesions found in reactive arthritis [Fig. 24.3]). Other individuals present with a septic joint,

TABLE 24.3. Differential diagnosis of reactive arthritis.

Gonococcal arthritis
Acute septic arthritis (excluding gonococcal arthritis)
Post-infectious arthritis:
- Post-streptococcal infection
- Lyme disease
- Viral arthritis, including rubella, Epstein–Barr virus, HIV, hepatitis B, and erythrovirus 19 (parvovirus)

Gout and pseudogout
Trauma
Psoriasis
Ankylosing spondylitis, ulcerative colitis and Crohn's disease
Behçet's disease
Sarcoidosis

FIGURE 24.2. Skin lesions of disseminated gonococcal infection.

with or without skin lesions. *Note*: Although DGI is most often associated with a septic joint, reactive arthritis is found in up to 20% of patients with gonorrhoea and arthritis.

Other than gonococcal arthritis, acute septic arthritis may be caused by numerous organisms, e.g., *Staphylococcus aureus, Streptococcus pyogenes, Neisseria meningitidis, Salmonella* spp., and *Streptococcus pneumoniae*. Any joint may become inflamed, but most often the knee, wrist, and elbow are affected.

In post-streptococcal infection, the onset of arthritis, which is usually polyarticular, is acute, when large joints are chiefly affected.

Borrelia burgdorferi is transmitted by the bite of an infected tick. Arthritis, which is usually episodic, develops weeks to months later, and principally affects the large joints. In this case, there is no history of exposure to ticks.

Acute episodes of gout usually affect a single peripheral joint, especially the first metatarsophalangeal joint. Pseudogout, acute synovitis associated with the deposition of calcium pyrophosphate crystals in articular cartilage, may resemble septic arthritis with fever. It is a condition found in the elderly and is an unlikely diagnosis here.

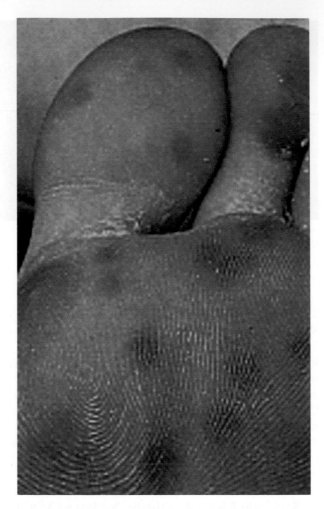

FIGURE 24.3. Pustular psoriasis (keratoderma blenorrhagica) of sole of foot.

Acute arthritis may be the presenting feature of ankylosing spondylitis, psoriatic arthritis, ulcerative colitis, Crohn's disease, Behçet's disease, but there are usually additional features of these conditions which are absent in this case.

Acute arthritis, often associated with erythema nodosum, may also be a feature of sarcoidosis.

A Gram-stained smear of urethral exudate shows about 20 polymorphonuclear leucocytes per ×1,000 microscopical field; Gram-negative diplococci are not seen. A urine sample contains large numbers of polymorphonuclear leucocytes but protein and red cells are absent. Urethral and pharyngeal material (taken as described in Case 1) is sent to the laboratory for culture for N. gon-orrhoeae, *and a first-voided specimen of urine is obtained for the detection of* C. trachomatis *by a nucleic acid amplification assay. A sample of synovial fluid, aspirated under aseptic conditions, appears yellow and turbid. Many polymorphonuclear leucocytes are seen on a Gram-stained smear of the aspirate, but neither Gram-positive nor Gram-negative bacteria are identified. Urate or pyrophosphate crystals are not seen in a sample examined by polarized light microscopy. An aliquot of fluid is sent for bacterial culture. The peripheral blood total white cell count is 14×10^9/L (normal range: $4.0–11.0 \times 10^9$/L), with a neutrophil leucocytosis; other hematological parameters are within normal limits. The erythrocyte sedimentation rate (ESR) is 75 mm/h (normally 0–10 mm/h), and the C-reactive protein concentration is 62 mg/L (normally <5 mg/L). Serum urate, calcium, and angiotensin-converting enzyme estimations are requested. Serum samples are also sent for the determination of anti-streptolysin O (ASO) and for rheumatoid factor. Serological tests for syphilis, Lyme disease, HIV, hepatitis B virus, Epstein–Barr virus, and erythrovirus 19 (parvovirus) are undertaken.*

How Do You Interpret These Laboratory Findings?

Although the leucocytosis, elevated ESR, and C-reactive protein indicate an acute inflammatory response, these changes are not specific.

The absence of Gram-negative diplococci in the urethral smear makes urethral gonorrhoea with dissemination an unlikely diagnosis. Culture from possibly infected anatomical sites (in this case, urethra and pharynx), as was performed in this case, however, is the investigation of choice for gonococcal arthritis. It should be noted that, as organisms are seldom visualized, failure to identify

Gram-negative diplococci in synovial fluid does not exclude the diagnosis.

Gram-smear microscopy of synovial fluid may aid in the diagnosis of non-gonococcal septic arthritis. Bacteria, however, are only visualized in about 50% of cases, but when detected Gram-positive and Gram-negative organisms can be differentiated, facilitating choice of initial antimicrobial therapy.

Failure to identify crystals in the synovial fluid makes a crystal arthropathy an unlikely diagnosis.

What Is the Most Likely Diagnosis and What Is the Initial Management?

The presumptive diagnosis is sexually acquired reactive arthritis (SARA), complicating probable urethral chlamydial infection. There is no history suggestive of intestinal infection, although some such infections are symptomless and difficult to detect by the time of development of arthritis.

Treatment is not curative but is aimed at relieving symptoms. When the patient first attends, the course of the disease should be fully explained to him. He should be told particularly that the acute episode may last for at least 6 weeks, but that sometimes it may last for much longer. The management of the features of SARA are as follows:

- The management of non-gonococcal urethritis has already been discussed (see Case 5). The presence of the complication of SARA does not alter the general approach. Treatment of the genital tract inflammation does not appear to alter the course of the disease.
- Conjunctivitis is a self-limiting condition, generally resolving within a few weeks of its onset. As anterior uveitis is a recognized complication of reactive arthritis, and may be difficult to recognize, referral to an ophthalmologist is recommended.
- During the acute stage of the illness, when the joints are markedly inflamed, bed rest is advisable. It is of great importance to ensure that the correct posture is assumed during this period of rest to reduce the risk of development of flexion defor-

mities. A physiotherapist can help with the patient's management. Non-steroidal anti-inflammatory drugs (NSAIDs), such as ibuprofen, are usually effective in the management of the arthritis of SARA. The aspiration of a tense effusion in the knee joint followed immediately by the instillation of a corticosteroid may be useful in alleviating joint symptoms.

- In the management of enthesitis, rest, physiotherapy, and ultrasound therapy are often helpful, but NSAIDs are also required. Local injection of a corticosteroid can give rapid relief of symptoms, but repeated injections may be necessary.
- Circinate balanitis (psoriasis of the penis) usually resolves spontaneously within a few weeks of its onset, but healing may be facilitated by the use of a topical steroid preparation, combined with an antimicrobial agent. When there is secondary bacterial infection, the use of local saline lavages, and dressings soaked in normal saline applied to the glans, are of value.

Five days after his clinic attendance, the laboratory test results are available. Chlamydia trachomatis *DNA was detected in the first-voided urine specimen, but* N. gonorrhoeae *was not isolated from the urethra or pharynx. Neither bacteria nor fungi were cultured from the synovial fluid. Serum urate, calcium, and angiotensin-converting enzyme concentrations were within normal limits, and serological tests for syphilis, Lyme disease, and the viral infections noted above were negative. The ASO titer was low.*

Have These Further Results Aided in the Diagnosis?

The detection of *C. trachomatis* in the urethra is further supporting evidence for a diagnosis of SARA. Negative urethral and pharyngeal cultures for *N. gonorrhoeae* effectively exclude a diagnosis of gonococcal arthritis. *Note*: Culture of joint aspirate for *N. gonorrhoeae* is positive in fewer than 50% of cases of gonococcal arthritis. Nevertheless, it is good practice to perform gonococcal culture on synovial fluid when the diagnosis of this condition is suspected.

As bacterial culture of synovial aspirate is positive in over 90% of cases of non-gonococcal septic arthritis, this diagnosis is very unlikely.

A normal serum urate concentration does not exclude gout, but the absence of urate crystals in the synovial fluid makes the diagnosis less likely.

In acute sarcoidosis, the serum calcium concentration is often, but not invariably elevated, as is that of angiotensin-converting enzyme. Normal concentrations in this case, and the absence of other clinical features such as erythema nodosum, make sarcoidosis an unlikely diagnosis.

The low concentration of anti-streptolysin O excludes a diagnosis of post-streptococcal infection, and the negative serological tests exclude Lyme disease, syphilis, and the viral infections associated with post-infectious arthritis.

The absence of associated features makes the diagnosis of ankylosing spondylitis, psoriatic arthritis, the arthritis associated with inflammatory bowel disease, and Behçet's disease less likely.

What Is the Course of SARA?

Sexually acquired reactive arthritis is a self-limiting condition. The duration of the first episode of SARA varies between 2 weeks and several years. In general (more than 70%) first episodes resolve within 12 weeks. At least half of patients develop recurrences, the interval between the initial episode and the recurrence varying between 3 months and up to 36 years. Although recurrence may be precipitated by urethritis or dysentery, other factors have been identified and include surgical operations on the urinary tract.

Following the acute arthritis of the initial episode, there may be no clinical evidence of joint damage. In some cases, with each recurrent episode of arthritis, permanent damage is done to the joint that may ultimately show the features of chronic arthritis. Uncommonly, in less than 5% of cases, following the initial episode of arthritis, resolution of the inflammatory process is incomplete and chronic arthritis rapidly develops in the affected joints. The patient complains of pain, stiffness, and swelling of the joint, the severity of symptoms being subject to exacerbations and remissions; deformity is the ultimate fate of joints affected in this way. Most frequently it is the joints of the lower limbs and the sacroiliac joints which bear the brunt of chronic arthritis in this disease. Generally, as chronic arthritis develops, other manifestations of the disease become less obvious, with the possible exception of anterior uveitis.

Case 25
A Woman with Recurrent Pruritus Vulvae

Two years later Margaret (Case 11) returns to the surgery. Over the past 18 months she has had at least ten episodes of vulval itch. She tells you that she has purchased both topical and oral antifungal preparations from her local pharmacist. Although these treatments have given some relief for a few weeks, nothing seems to "fix my problem permanently." She is still using the combined contraceptive pill and has had no pregnancies. Her husband is symptomless.

What Would You Do Next?

In the first instance, it is important to confirm the diagnosis of recurrent candidiasis, as other conditions can mimic this infection (see Case 11). At this consultation she is symptomless and you establish that she has not used potential irritants or allergens before the onset of the pruritus.

You examine her for lesions suggestive of genital dermatoses, but the vulva appears normal and the vaginal mucosa is healthy.

At this stage it is pointless to culture for *Candida* spp., as these fungi are often present in the normal vagina, and a positive culture cannot tell if her symptoms are indeed attributable to candidiasis.

You invite her to attend the surgery should symptoms recur and before she has taken any treatment.

Margaret returns 2 weeks later. The vulval irritation had recurred the day previously. You find marked vulval erythema; the walls of the vagina are inflamed, and there are white adherent plaques (Fig. 25.1). You think the appearance is that of candidiasis, but you wish to confirm the diagnosis. How is this done?

A specimen of vaginal material is taken with a cotton wool-tipped applicator stick and sent to the laboratory in the appropriate transport medium (for example, Amies'). Some of the material is

A. McMillan, *Sexually Transmissible Infections in Clinical Practice*, 167
DOI 10.1007/978-1-84882-557-4_25,
© Springer-Verlag London Limited 2009

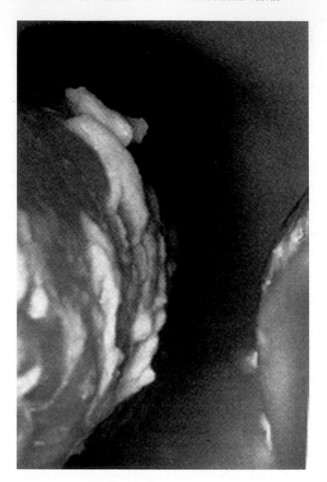

FIGURE 25.1. White plaques adherent to vaginal wall.

emulsified in a drop of potassium hydroxide solution and examined
microscopically for fungi. Alternatively, a Gram-stained smear is
prepared and examined for the Gram-positive fungal hyphae, pseudohyphae, or spores (Fig. 25.2). [1]

---

[1] All pathogenic *Candida* species multiply by the production of buds from
a thin-walled ovoid *blastospore* (yeast cell). A *hypha* is a long micro-

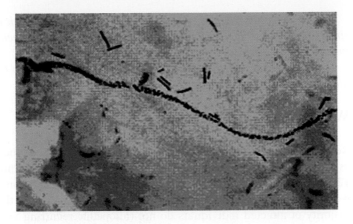

FIGURE 25.2. Pseudohypha of *Candida albicans*.

Although budding yeasts may be seen, hyphae are not a feature of infection with *C. glabrata*, a fungus that is becoming more common as a cause of vaginal candidiasis and that has reduced susceptibility to the azole antifungal drugs. Other species of *Candida* that may infect the vagina include *C. parapsilosis*, *C. tropicalis*, and *C. krusei*; the majority of these fungi show reduced susceptibility to azole antifungal drugs.

Although culture with speciation of the isolate is not generally undertaken in the management of women with acute candidal vulvovaginitis, recurrent disease may be associated with *Candida* species with reduced susceptibility to azoles (see Case 26), and in these cases, such testing is warranted. Antifungal susceptibility testing of *C. albicans* isolated from women with recurrent vulvovaginitis is rarely helpful.

---

scopic tube made up of multiple fungal cell units divided by septa. Hyphae arise as branches of existing hyphae or by the germination of spores. A *pseudohypha* arises by a budding process in which each generation of buds remains attached to its parent; the buds of the first and subsequent generations are narrow elongated cells that do not resemble the parent blastospore. The end-to-end aggregation of elongated blastoconidia or pseudohypha are distinguished from true *hyphae* in that there are constrictions at the septal junctions.

Having taken the vaginal specimen, you treat Margaret with a single oral dose of fluconazole and invite her to return in 2 weeks time when the laboratory results will be available.

You subsequently receive the report that shows infection with C. albicans.

What Treatment Would You Offer Margaret?

Recurrent vulvovaginal candidiasis (RVVC) may be defined as four episodes of mycologically proven candidiasis within 12 months and affects fewer than 5% of women. Although some women have recognizable factors that predispose to RVVC, the majority of affected individuals do not (idiopathic recurring vulvovaginitis). For many years it was proposed that the condition represented re-infection either from the gastrointestinal tract or from a sexual partner. This theory has now been abandoned in favor of one that suggests that organisms are not completely eliminated by treatment and that patients have relapsing vaginitis as a result of a change in the normal protective host defense mechanisms. The finding that the identical strain type of *C albicans* causes most sequential episodes and that very high re-colonization rates are found within 1 month of a short-term therapy supports this hypothesis.

Reductions in local immune responses, however, are more likely to be important in pathogenesis.

Good clinical trials of treatment for this distressing condition are lacking and guidelines are empirical. When the diagnosis is established, treatment is initiated with any of the antifungal preparations noted above, as you have already done. (Either vaginal preparations or oral azoles may be used, but, as the response to single-dose therapy with the latter is sometimes unsatisfactory, a course of therapy lasting for 7–14 days should be given [fluconazole should be prescribed as a 50 mg capsule, given orally once daily]. When vaginal pessaries or intra-vaginal cream is used, cream should also be applied to the vulval skin.) Maintenance treatment is initiated immediately after resolution of symptoms. This may be with

1. vaginal pessaries, such as *clotrimazole* 500 mg used once weekly or
2. oral *fluconazole* 150 mg, given once weekly.

The length of treatment must be tailored to the individual patient, but is unlikely to be less than 6 months. At the end of this period it is worth discontinuing therapy to assess outcome. Further therapy may be necessary.

There is no evidence that treatment of the sexual partner influences recurrence.

Case 26
A Woman with Pruritus Vulvae (2)

Margaret (Case 11 and 24) returns to the Sexual Health clinic 6 years later with a 4 week history of vulval itch. Although she has had no recurrences of candidiasis for 3 years, she thought that candidiasis was the most likely cause of her symptoms and she self-medicated with oral fluconazole and topical clotrimazole, obtained over the counter from a pharmacy. Her symptoms, however, remain unchanged and she consults you for advice. When you examine her, the findings are similar to those described previously, but you decide to send a specimen of vaginal discharge to the laboratory to confirm the diagnosis.

A Gram-stained smear shows many blastospores but no hyphae (Fig. 26.1).

What Is the Most Likely Diagnosis, and What Is Your Immediate Management?

The finding of blastospores without hyphae suggests infection with *C. glabrata*. The clinical response of *C. glabrata*, the second most common isolate from women with recurrent vulvovaginal candidiasis, to topical or oral antifungal agents may be unsatisfactory. The minimum inhibitory concentrations (MICs) of the available azoles are generally higher for *C. glabrata* than for *C albicans*, and in many cases, there is frank resistance to fluconazole. Itraconazole has moderate activity against *C. glabrata*, but the MIC for the isolate does not always predict therapeutic success. In the treatment of vulvovaginal candidiasis caused by *C glabrata* itraconazole in an oral dosage of 200 mg twice daily for 7 days is the treatment of choice. If oral fluconazole or miconazole are used, prolonged

A. McMillan, *Sexually Transmissible Infections in Clinical Practice*, 173
DOI 10.1007/978-1-84882-557-4_26,
© Springer-Verlag London Limited 2009

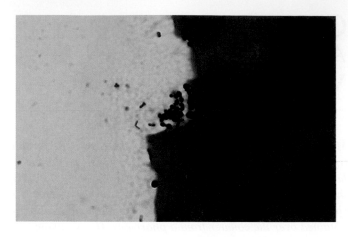

FIGURE 26.1. Blastospores adherent to epithelial cells.

courses are usually necessary; shorter courses or single-dose therapy should be avoided.

The mycology laboratory confirms that the infecting species is Candida glabrata. *If itraconazole treatment fails to achieve cure, what other treatments might you consider?*

When azole treatment of recurrent vulvovaginitis caused by *C. glabrata* has failed, boric acid (in a capsule containing 600 mg) inserted into the vagina once daily for 14 days has resulted in mycological cure rates of about 75%. If this treatment is successful, maintenance therapy in the form of nystatin pessaries, inserted into the vagina nightly, should be instituted. Maintenance therapy with boric acid (600 mg twice weekly) has also been used with some success. Prolonged absorption of boric acid, however, may cause systemic toxic effects such as anorexia, weight loss, skin rashes, and anemia, and its use should be confined to specialists. The safety of boric acid in pregnancy is uncertain, and it is recommended that its use should be discontinued 1–2 weeks before conception.

Amphotericin B 50 mg suppositories, one inserted into the vagina nightly for 14 nights has resulted in cure of about 70% of patients treated for vulvovaginal infection with non-*albicans* candidal infection. The treatment has been well tolerated.

Intra-vaginal flucytosine cream (17%) instilled nightly for 14 nights has also been used in the treatment of azole-resistant candidal infections, but this drug is not readily available, and experience in is use is very limited. There is also concern that drug resistance may rapidly develop.

Case 27
A Young Woman with Abdominal Pain

Amanda, a 21-year-old student, attends a Sexual Health clinic because her boyfriend had been diagnosed as having urethral chlamydial infection 2 days previously. She tells you that for the past 2 weeks she has had intermittent lower abdominal discomfort, particularly on the right side. She also complains of persistent pain in the right upper abdomen, the pain radiating intermittently to the right shoulder, and being exacerbated by deep inspiration. Her periods have been regular, the most recent having been 14 days previously, and had been normal. She has not noticed increased vaginal discharge, but she has had some vaginal bleeding during the past week. There are no urinary or gastrointestinal symptoms. She has been in a regular relationship for 3 months, and she had had unprotected vaginal intercourse with her partner 2 days prior to her clinic attendance. Over the preceding 3 weeks she has had lower abdominal pain during intercourse. For 5 years she has used the combined oral contraceptive, and she has not missed any pills in the recent past. Her general health has been good, and she has not had any serious illnesses in the past.

What Conditions Would You Consider as Causes of Her Abdominal Symptoms?

Amanda is a known sexual contact of a man with chlamydiae, and it is highly likely that she will also be infected. A common complication of chlamydial infection in women is pelvic inflammatory disease (PID) – an estimated 10% of infected women develop PID – and the history is compatible with this diagnosis. Pain in the right upper abdomen may be a manifestation of perihepatitis

A. McMillan, *Sexually Transmissible Infections in Clinical Practice*, 177
DOI 10.1007/978-1-84882-557-4_27,
© Springer-Verlag London Limited 2009

(Fitz–Hugh–Curtis syndrome), resulting from chlamydiae tracking from the uterine tubes to the liver capsule.

Other conditions, however, need to be considered (see Case 14, Table 14.1). Acute appendicitis, mesenteric lymphadenitis, and regional ileitis can produce right-sided lower abdominal pain, and, of course, ectopic pregnancy has to be excluded. The absence of urinary symptoms speaks against urinary tract infection or ureteric calculus. Pain in the right hypochondrium may result from acute cholecystitis, or from right-sided pleurisy.

Amanda looks distressed and in considerable abdominal pain. Her temperature is 37.5° C, and her pulse rate 90 per minute. There are no abnormal chest findings. The abdomen moves with respiration. She is tender over the right hypochondrium but the liver is not palpable. There is tenderness with rebound in the right but not the left iliac fossa. Bowel sounds are present, but a friction rub is not heard over the right hypochondrium. The cervix appears normal, and pain is not elicited when it is moved. There is minimal tenderness in the right but not in the left fornix; the uterine tubes cannot be felt, and there are no pelvic masses. A pregnancy test on a urine sample is negative. Gram-smear microscopy of endocervical material shows numerous polymorphonuclear leucocytes but no Gram-negative diplococci.

The hemoglobin concentration in the peripheral blood is 118 g/L, the total white cell count is 9.9 × 10^9/L, and the polymorphonuclear count is 8.2 × 10^9/L. The erythrocyte sedimentation rate (ESR) is 90 mm. The plasma bilirubin concentration and plasma enzyme tests of liver function are normal.

Do the Clinical and Laboratory Findings Aid the Differential Diagnosis?

Although a negative pregnancy test does not rule out ectopic pregnancy, this is an unlikely diagnosis because she had a normal period some 14 days previously, she uses oral contraception consistently, and a mass is not found on pelvic examination. The most likely diagnosis remains PID with perihepatitis. However, the predominantly right-sided abdominal pain with minimal pelvic tenderness raises the possibility that she has acute appendicitis. Laparoscopy is therefore arranged.

Fibrinous adhesions between the liver, diaphragm, and anterior abdominal wall were found. The uterine tubes appeared normal.

The laparoscopic findings confirm the diagnosis of perihepatitis, most likely caused by chlamydiae. Indeed a subsequent report from the microbiology laboratory confirmed that *Chlamydia trachomatis* had been identified in endocervical specimen taken on the day of her clinic attendance; nucleic acid amplification assay for *Neisseria gonorrhoeae* yielded negative results.

Laparoscopy is not a routine investigation in women with suspected PID. If there is doubt about the diagnosis, in particular if a surgical emergency cannot be ruled out from the clinical findings as in this case, however, laparoscopy is a useful tool. The tubes may appear edematous and reddened, and exudate may be seen on the tubal surface. In early PID, the inflammatory reaction in the tubes may not extend to the serosal surface, and therefore the tubes may appear normal at laparoscopy. This may explain the finding in this case.

Amanda is treated with ofloxacin and metronidazole (see Case 14, *Table 14.3) and is reviewed 72 h after initiation of therapy. Her abdominal pain has improved considerably, and she is tolerating the antimicrobial regimen well.*

It is recommended that patients with PID are reviewed 4 weeks after therapy to ensure that the clinical response has been satisfactory and that partner notification has been completed.

Case 28
Gonococcal and Chlamydial Infections in a Pregnant Woman

Sarah, a 17-year-old woman, who is 14 weeks' pregnant attends a Sexual Health clinic as a sexual contact of a man with proven urethral gonorrhoea and chlamydial infection. She has noticed some increased vaginal discharge, but she is otherwise symptomless. For the past 6 months she has been in a relationship with the man who is her first and only sexual partner. He had had unprotected oral and vaginal sex with a woman from London about 3 weeks previously, and he had vaginal intercourse with Sarah 1 week later. At that time he was symptomless. She has documented hypersensitivity to penicillin, having had an anaphylactic reaction after receiving penicillin for the treatment of a dog bite several years previously.

Increased vaginal discharge is common during pregnancy and this symptom does not necessarily indicate infection. There is a high probability, however, that she is infected.

Specimens for culture for Neisseria gonorrhoeae *are obtained from the urethra, endocervical canal, anorectum, and pharynx, and endocervical material is taken for the detection of* Chlamydia trachomatis *(see Case 2). Gram-smear microscopy of urethral and endocervical material shows many polymorphonuclear leucocytes but Gram-negative diplococci are not identified. Microscopy of a saline-mount preparation of vaginal material does not show* Trichomonas vaginalis. *Tests for treponemal and HIV infections are taken.*

Sarah is offered and accepts empirical treatment.

The reasons for this decision to offer empirical treatment for gonococcal and chlamydial infections are outlined in Cases 6 and 8.

A. McMillan, *Sexually Transmissible Infections in Clinical Practice*,   181
DOI 10.1007/978-1-84882-557-4_28,
© Springer-Verlag London Limited 2009

TABLE 28.1. Antimicrobial susceptibility results.

Antimicrobial agent	Interpretation of susceptibility result
Penicillin	Resistant
Tetracycline	Sensitive
Ciprofloxacin	Sensitive
Azithromycin	Sensitive
Spectinomycin	Sensitive
Ceftriaxone	Sensitive
Cefixime	Sensitive

Table 28.1 shows the results of the antimicrobial susceptibility testing of the Neisseria gonorrhoeae *isolated from her partner's urethra.*

What Would Be Your Choice of Antimicrobial Agent(s) in This Case?

Consider first the treatment of gonorrhoea in a pregnant woman. Tetracyclines and the quinolones are contraindicated in pregnancy.

Although the cephalosporins ceftriaxone and cefixime are highly active against *N. gonorrhoeae*, there is concern about the administration of these drugs to individuals with a documented history of penicillin hypersensitivity. About 8% of persons with penicillin allergy show hypersensitivity reactions when given a cephalosporin. Skin testing for cephalosporin hypersensitivity may identify those who are unlikely to develop a serious reaction, but such tests have not been fully standardized and are not generally available.

As azithromycin is useful in the treatment of genital chlamydial infection that is commonly found in association with gonorrhoea, it is tempting to consider this agent. There are, however, concerns about its use. Although a 2 g single oral dose of azithromycin has been shown to be effective in the treatment of gonorrhoea, this dose[1] results in a high incidence of gastrointestinal side effects. The emergence of resistant strains of *N. gonorrhoeae* is of concern, and, although the infecting strain appears sensitive to azithromycin in vitro, this may not accurately reflect efficacy in the clinical situation.

Spectinomycin, given as a single intramuscular injection of 2 g, is the treatment of choice in this case. It is highly effective against *N. gonorrhoeae* has few side effects and is safe to use in pregnancy.

Treatment of probable concurrent chlamydial infection needs to be considered.

Although azithromycin appears to be safe and many clinicians prescribe it for the treatment of chlamydial infection, it is not licensed for use in pregnancy, and current UK guidelines recommend its use only when there are no satisfactory alternatives. In a meta-analysis of randomized controlled trials, single-dose azithromycin was shown to be as effective as a course of erythromycin in the treatment of pregnant women but was associated with fewer adverse events. Table 28.2 indicates the antimicrobial agents that are currently recommended for use in pregnant women with chlamydial genital tract infection.

TABLE 28.2. Antimicrobial drugs recommended for use in pregnant women with chlamydial genital tract infection.

Erythromycin 500 mg four times daily by mouth for 7 days

OR

Erythromycin 500 mg twice daily by mouth for 14 days

OR

Amoxicillin 500 mg three times per day for 7 days

---

[1] A single oral dose of 1 g of azithromycin is used for the treatment of genital chlamydial infection. This dose, however, has not been shown to be very effective in the treatment of gonorrhoea.

Sarah is treated with spectinomycin and erythromycin, given in an oral dose of 500 mg twice daily. She is invited to attend the clinic 1 week later.

At this time the results of the microbiological tests are available:

- *Neisseria gonorrhoeae* was isolated from the urethra, endocervical canal, and anorectum but not from the pharynx. The antimicrobial susceptibility pattern of the isolate was identical to that of her partner's.
- *Chlamydia trachomatis* DNA was detected in the endocervical sample.
- Serological tests for syphilis and HIV were negative.

She has not had sexual contact since initiation of treatment.

The reason for review at this time is to ensure that the treatment regimen is well tolerated and that there has been no risk of re-infection. As she has been treated with a drug to which the infecting strain is sensitive, this has been given under supervision, and there is no apparent risk of re-infection, a test of cure for gonorrhoea is not indicated.[2]

As efficacy of treatment of genital chlamydial infection in pregnant women with any of the drugs listed in Table 28.2   (and of azithromycin) is thought to be <95%, a test of cure should be undertaken (at least 5 weeks after completion of therapy if a nucleic acid amplification assay is used).

What Are the Risks of Untreated Gonococcal and Chlamydial Infections in Pregnant Women?

(a) *Gonococcal infection.*

In pregnant women, untreated gonorrhoea is associated with an increased risk of

---

[2]If a test of cure is undertaken, this should be performed at least 72 h after completion of antimicrobial therapy. As cure of infection of the pharynx is less certain than infection of the genital tract or anorectum, at least one test of cure should be performed if gonorrhoea is identified at this anatomical site.

- Chorioamnionitis;
- Intrauterine growth retardation;
- Premature rupture of the membranes ;
- Pre-maturity;
- Low birth weight;
- Fetal death;
- Post-partum PID;
- Post-termination endometritis;
- Disseminated gonococcal infection in the mother (see Case 24). Pregnancy is a predisposing factor to dissemination, particularly during the third trimester.

Neisseria gonorrhoeae can also be transmitted to the neonate during vaginal delivery and result in ophthalmia neonatorum (Fig. 28.1). The risk of transmission from an infected mother is estimated to be between 30 and 50%. Most infants develop conjunctivitis within 24–48 h of birth. The eyelids swell and pus collects in the conjunctival sac. Keratitis with corneal scarring may result if the condition is not treated.

(b) *Chlamydial infection.*

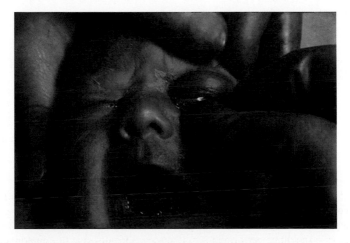

FIGURE 28.1. Gonococcal ophthalmia neonatorum.

Untreated chlamydial infection may be associated with the following:

- Premature rupture of the membranes and premature delivery, although the evidence is inconclusive.
- Neonatal transmission. About 75% of infants delivered vaginally to infected mothers, and just over 20% born by Caesarean section to infected women with intact membranes become infected. The latter finding suggests that infection in utero is possible. Conjunctivitis, developing 3–13 days after birth, and varying in severity from mild to severe, is the most obvious clinical presentation of chlamydial neonatal infection. In the absence of specific treatment, the course is usually benign. The sight is not compromised, although micropannus and conjunctival scarring may occur. Infection is not confined to the conjunctiva, and the respiratory tract, the middle ear, the gut, and the vagina can be also become infected. Spread of the organism from the nasopharynx to the lower respiratory tract can result in pneumonitis, with an estimated incidence of 11–20% of babies born to infected mothers. The onset of the pneumonitis occurs later than that of conjunctivitis, usually between 3 and 11 weeks. The infection is generally mild and self-limiting, but treatment in the form of erythromycin is often advocated.

Case 29
A Pregnant Woman with Genital Herpes

Samantha is a 28-year-old woman who presents to a Sexual Health clinic with a 3 day history of painful swelling and ulceration of the vulva. She has felt unwell with fever for a few days. She is 37 weeks pregnant to her husband who has a history of recurrent genital herpes. They had unprotected sexual intercourse about 1 week before the onset of her symptoms; her husband had no obvious signs of recurrent herpes at that time. Physical examination confirms the presence of multiple ulcers on the labia majora, labia minora, and at the introitus (Fig. 29.1). She also has bilateral tender inguinal lymph node enlargement.

How Would You Manage This Case?

Samantha should be treated with either oral or intravenous aciclovir (see Case 16 for information on oral aciclovir).

Herpes simplex virus can be transmitted to the neonate from a mother with primary or initial genital herpes at term. It has been estimated that the risk of neonatal herpes developing after vaginal delivery to a mother with primary or initial genital herpes simplex virus (HSV) infection is about 40%. The neonate may develop disseminated infection, affecting particularly the liver and adrenal glands, or localized infection affecting the central nervous system, eye, skin, or oral cavity. The mortality rate for infants with disseminated or central nervous system disease is high.

Mothers with symptomatic primary or initial herpes at term or within 6 weeks of expected delivery should be delivered by Caesarean section before the membranes have ruptured or within 4 h of their rupture. Performing a Caesarean section beyond this time is not likely to protect the fetus. If vaginal delivery is

A. McMillan, *Sexually Transmissible Infections in Clinical Practice*,   187
DOI 10.1007/978-1-84882-557-4_29,
© Springer-Verlag London Limited 2009

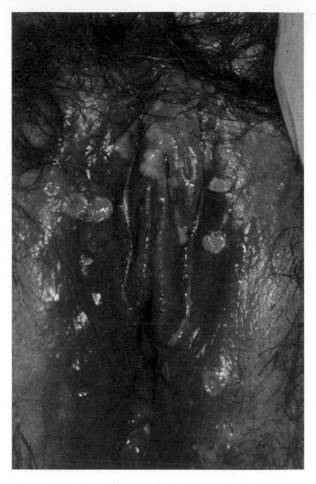

FIGURE 29.1. Multiple vulval ulcers in a pregnant woman.

performed, or if the membranes have been ruptured for more than 4 h, the mother should be treated intra-partum, and subsequently the neonate with intravenous aciclovir. Vaginal procedures such as the application of scalp electrodes are best avoided to reduce the risk of damaging the baby's skin and allowing viral entry. There should be consultation with a pediatrician.

Note: Primary or initial genital herpes during the first or second trimester should be treated as in the non-pregnant patient (see Case 16). As developmental abnormalities have not been associated with HSV infection, termination of pregnancy is not indicated. Although aciclovir is not licensed for use in pregnancy, there has now been substantial use of the drug by pregnant women, and, in keeping with the results of tests on animals, there has been no evidence of teratogenicity.

Two years later, Samantha who is 3 months pregnant with her second child attends the clinic for advice on the management of symptomatic recurrences during her pregnancy. She also asks if it is necessary to deliver this child by Caesarean section.

What Advice Would You Give?

Symptomatic recurrences even in pregnant women are likely to be of short duration, and drug therapy is usually unnecessary. If the episodes are severe, however, episodic treatment with aciclovir may be offered.

The risk of transmission of HSV from a woman with recurrent genital herpes to a child at the time of delivery is low. Caesarean section is only recommended for those with lesions at term. There are now good data to show that the prophylactic use of aciclovir or valaciclovir reduces the likelihood of clinical recurrence at the time of delivery and the need for Caesarean section. For this reason, aciclovir, in a dosage of 400 mg three times per day[1] by mouth may be offered to women with a history of recurrent genital herpes who wish to avoid delivery by Caesarean section. Treatment should be initiated at 36 weeks' gestation.

---

[1]The higher dose of aciclovir has been recommended because of the altered pharmacokinetics during late pregnancy (2007 National Guideline for the Management of Genital Herpes).

Case 30
A Pregnant Woman with Genital Warts

Linda (Case 15), a 22-year-old woman, is referred to a Sexual Health clinic by an obstetrician. She is 16 weeks pregnant and has noticed lumps appearing on her genitals. She has had the same sexual partner for 5 years and neither has had sexual contact with other individuals. Examination shows multiple warts on the labia majora, labia minora, and at the introitus (Fig. 30.1).

She is very concerned (a) about the effect of the warts on the pregnancy, (b) about treatment, (c) will it be necessary to deliver the baby by Caesarean section, and (d) that the child will be born with or subsequently develop warts. She also wants to know how she could have acquired the warts.

What Do You Tell Her?

(a) Human papillomavirus infection is not associated with adverse outcomes of pregnancy such as pre-term birth, low birth weight, and premature rupture of the membranes. The presence of genital warts is not an indication for termination of pregnancy.

(b) In pregnant women, spontaneous regression of condylomata acuminata warts often occurs during the first few weeks after delivery. During the pregnancy, when the lesions are small and symptomless, a non-intervention approach is reasonable. The woman should be reassured that spontaneous regression within several weeks of delivery is the usual outcome and that any persistent warts can be treated as described in Case 15. There is no evidence that eradication of warts during pregnancy reduces the risk of perinatal transmission which, in any case, is low (see below). In some cases, for example, when

A. McMillan, *Sexually Transmissible Infections in Clinical Practice*, 191
DOI 10.1007/978-1-84882-557-4_30,
© Springer-Verlag London Limited 2009

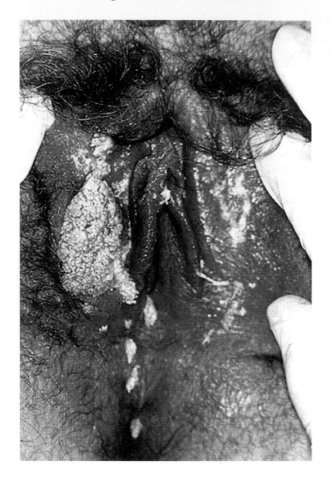

FIGURE 30.1. Vulval warts in a pregnant woman.

warts become large, bleed easily, and become uncomfortable, or from patient choice, treatment is indicated. Options, however, are somewhat limited. The use of podophyllotoxin should be avoided, and the safety of imiquimod in pregnancy has not been established. Scissor excision of extensive lesions may result in severe hemorrhage and diathermy may cause considerable post-operative pain. Cryotherapy, electrocautery, or the cautious application of trichloroethanoic acid can be used to treat small condylomata but recurrence or persistence is common during the pregnancy. Laser vaporization yields good results, but when warts are extensive, general anesthesia is required.

(c) As the risks of surgery are likely to outweigh the possible benefits of reducing the risk of perinatal transmission of HPV to the neonate, Caesarean section is not indicated in the management of women with genital warts except in the rare instances when they are so large that they obstruct labor or are thought likely to cause significant hemorrhage during vaginal delivery.

(d) Mother-to-child transmission of HPV can result in

- *Juvenile-onset respiratory papillomatosis.* This condition is almost always associated with infection with HPV types 6/11, and a maternal history of genital warts is a strong risk factor. As affected children have been born to mothers delivered by Caesarean section, it is probable that some infants become infected through ascending infection. The prevalence of the condition is unknown, but in a Danish study of children born to mothers with a history of genital warts, 7 of 1000 children developed respiratory papillomatosis. Juvenile-onset disease usually presents between 3 months and 5 years of birth. Hoarseness is the usual feature. Papillomata develop on the laryngeal surface of the epiglottis, the upper and lower margins of the ventricles, the under-surface of the vocal cords and the carina, less commonly, the distal trachea and bronchi. Untreated, there is progressive respiratory obstruction with stridor, and possibly death.

- *Anogenital warts.* These may develop in children born to mothers with a history of genital warts. The prevalence is unknown, but the risk of neonatal infection with HPV appears to be low. A child can become infected in utero, or, during parturition. The pre-patent period is difficult to assess, but some clinicians consider an upper limit of 2 to 3 years from birth.

The appearance of genital warts during pregnancy does not necessarily indicate infidelity. Under hormonal influence, HPV is up-regulated in pregnancy, and as a result, latent virus, possibly acquired years previously, may become apparent.

Case 31
A Gay Man with Diarrhea

Samuel, a 24-year-old British, man attends a Gay Man's Sexual Health clinic for investigation of troublesome diarrhea. For the preceding 10 days he has been passing loose watery stools about five times per day. The stools are offensive, float on the surface of the water in the toilet, and are difficult to flush away. He has not, however, noticed blood, pus, or mucus in the stools. His appetite has been poor, and he has had some upper abdominal discomfort with increased flatulence. He is otherwise symptomless, in particular he has not felt feverish. He has not traveled outwith the United Kingdom within the past 2 years. There is no past history of gastrointestinal disorders. He has been fully immunized against hepatitis A and B.

In the past 3 months he has had about 15 different and unknown male sexual partners. He has had protected receptive and insertive anal intercourse with six of these men, but he has had unprotected oral–genital and oral–anal sex with each man. His most recent sexual contact had been about 14 days prior to the clinic attendance.

What Sexually Transmissible Infections Would You Consider in the Differential Diagnosis?

Sexually transmissible infections can cause a variety of intestinal disorders, particularly among men who have sex with men (MSM), as shown in Table 31.1. Bacteria such as *Neisseria gonorrhoeae*, *Chlamydia trachomatis*, and herpes simplex virus can be transmitted by receptive anal intercourse and cause distal proctitis. Oral–anal sex (*rimming*) can result in the acquisition of organisms

A. McMillan, *Sexually Transmissible Infections in Clinical Practice*,   195
DOI 10.1007/978-1-84882-557-4_31,
© Springer-Verlag London Limited 2009

TABLE 31.1 Sexually transmissible causes of enteropathy, proctocolitis, and distal proctitis.

Causes of enteropathy	Causes of proctocolitis	Causes of distal proctitis
Giardia intestinalis	*Shigella* spp.	*Neisseria gonorrhoeae*
Cryptosporidium spp.	*Campylobacter* spp.	*Chlamydia trachomatis:* Genotype A–K
Enterotoxigenic *Escherichia coli*	*Salmonella* spp.	Genotype L (LGV[a])
	Entamoeba histolytica	*Treponema pallidum*
Rotaviruses[c]		
	Cryptosporidium spp.	Herpes simplex virus
Group F adenoviruses[c]		
	Cytomegalovirus[b]	
Small-round-structured viruses[c]		

[a]LGV = lymphogranuloma venereum.
[b]In severely immunocompromised patients (in the context of HIV infection, CD4$^+$ T-cell count <100/mm^3).[1]
[c]Sexual transmission possible but not yet described in the literature.

transmissible by the fecal–oral route and shown in Table 30.1 as possible causes of enteropathy and proctocolitis.

The clinical features are not those of a distal proctitis (see Case 20), in which constipation is a more likely symptom than diarrhea, and in the absence of blood, pus, and mucus in the stools, proctocolitis is unlikely. Small intestinal infection with *Giardia intestinalis* or *Cryptosporidium* spp., however, is a possible cause of this man's symptoms. The pre-patent periods of giardiasis and cryptosporidium infections are estimated to be between 12 and 19 days, and 1–14 days, respectively. Self-limiting diarrhea may also be a feature of primary HIV infection, occurring on average about 14 days after infection. There are, however, usually associated symptoms such as fever, sore throat, swollen lymph glands, arthral-gia, and a skin rash. Rotaviruses, adenoviruses, particularly Group F, and small-round-structured viruses can be transmitted by the fecal–oral route, and MSM who practice oral–anal sex may there-fore be at risk. The pre-patent period of acute viral gastroenteritis is short – usually 1–2 days, but sometimes up to 7 days in the case of rotavirus and adenovirus infection – and the diarrhea usually lasts for less than 1 week. This diagnosis is therefore unlikely.

Samuel looks well, with no evidence of weight loss. His temper-ature is 36.5°C. There is no skin rash, and the mouth and pharynx appear normal. Significant enlargement of the superficial lymph nodes is not found. The abdomen moves well with respiration, and there is no tenderness or guarding. There are no abdominal masses, and neither the liver nor spleen is palpable. The perianal region is normal. Anoscopy shows watery stool in the lumen of the rectum whose mucosa appears normal; the vascular pattern is nor-mal, the mucosa does not bleed easily, and mucopus is not noted in the lumen.

Do the Clinical Findings Help Narrow the Differential Diagnosis?

There is no evidence of distal proctitis, but the clinical findings support the conclusion that he has an enteropathy.

Microbiological tests for gonococcal, chlamydial, treponemal, and HIV infections are undertaken as described in Case 4, *and a stool sample is obtained for microbiological investigation, includ-ing parasitology.*

Samuel attends the clinic 1 week later. His symptoms remain unchanged. The tests undertaken at the initial attendance yielded negative results for N. gonorrhoeae, C. trachomatis, Shigella *spp.,* Campylobacter *spp.,* Salmonella *spp., and enterotoxigenic* Escherichia coli. *Neither trophozoites nor cysts of* G. intestinalis *were detected by microscopy, and oocysts of Cryptosporidium spp. were not seen in a stained preparation of the stool sample. Serological tests for syphilis, including an anti-treponemal IgM*

*enzyme immunoassay (EIA), were negative, and a combined anti-
gen/antibody EIA for HIV was also negative.*

How Do You Interpret the Results of the Parasitological Investigations?

The absence of trophozoites or cysts of *G. intestinalis* in a single stool sample does not exclude infection with this protozoan. Multiple stool samples (at least three) should be tested before a negative result is reported. Direct immunofluorescence and immunoassays that have high sensitivity, specificity, positive, and negative predictive values when compared with the standard microscopical diagnostic methods have become available commercially. They are generally considered to be more sensitive than microscopy. False negative results in the antigen detection methods, however, may result when there are low parasite numbers, and repeat testing is recommended when a negative result is obtained but the diagnosis is strongly suspected. These tests may remain positive for some time after the parasite has been cleared. Some commercially available assays provide for the simultaneous detection of *Giardia* and *Cryptosporidium*.

A further three stool samples were sent to the laboratory. Cysts of G. intestinalis *are found in the third specimen. Oocysts of* Cryptosporidium *spp. were not detected, and culture of these specimens yielded negative results for bacterial pathogens.*

Giardia intestinalis (also known as *G. lamblia* or *G. duodenalis*) is an intestinal flagellated protozoan. The trophozoite (Fig. 31.1) is pear shaped, and the ventral surface is modified into an adhesive disc by which it attaches to the epithelium of the duodenum and jejunum. There are two oval nuclei and eight flagella. The trophozoites multiply by binary fission. Some pass down the small intestine and encyst. It is the cyst (Fig. 31.2) that is the infective stage. Cysts are passed out in the feces, and, after ingestion by the host, they excyst shortly after entering the upper small intestine. Two small trophozoites emerge from the cyst, divide, and become normal trophozoites.

Giardiasis is an infection found in both temperate and tropical countries, particularly where sanitation is poor. It is estimated

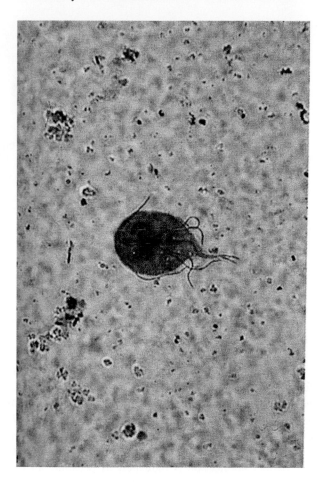

FIGURE 31.1. Trophozoite of *Giardia intestinalis*.

that 10–100 cysts are required to initiate infection (more than 300×10^6 cysts may be found in 1 mL of feces from some symptomatic patients). The infection is acquired by the ingestion of cysts in food or drink, and by direct fecal spread from one person to another. In the context of sexual transmission, oral–anal intercourse is probably important. Many infections are symptomless and transient, but in other individuals diarrhea results and

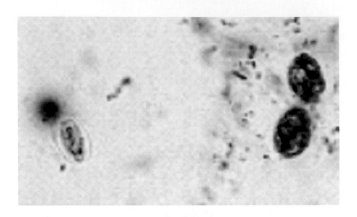

FIGURE 31.2. Cysts of *Giardia intestinalis.*

malabsorption may be a feature. Untreated, symptoms usually resolve after a variable interval of up to 3 months.

How Would You Treat Samuel?

Table 31.2   indicates recommended treatment regimens for giardiasis.

Samuel is treated with metronidazole 2 g daily by mouth for 3 days. He is warned about the interaction between the alcohol and the drug (see Case 10). What further action would you advise?

As it is probable that Samuel acquired *Giardia* through sexual contact, partner notification is indicated. If possible, all partners

TABLE 31.2 Recommended treatment regimes for giardiasis.

Metronidazole 2 g once daily by mouth for 3 days
OR
Metronidazole 400 mg three times per day by mouth for 5 days
OR
Tinidazole 2 g as a single oral dose

within the preceding month should be screened for symptomatic infection, and treated if necessary. After treatment, three stool samples, taken not less than 24 h apart should be obtained to confirm cure. In some patients, intestinal symptoms may persist for several weeks after eradication of infection. This is attributed to slow recovery of function of the intestinal epithelium.

Case 32
A Gay Man with Jaundice

Michael, a 19-year-old man, presents to his General Practitioner with a 7-day history of nausea, malaise, poor appetite, and discomfort in the right upper abdomen. Over the past few days he has noticed that his urine is darker than normal and that his stools are pale. His friends have told him that his skin looks yellowish. He drinks about 10 units of alcohol per week, but he does not use recreational drugs, and he is not receiving any medication. He has not traveled abroad in the past 2 years. He lives with his parents and a 16-year-old sister. For the past 3 months Michael has been in a regular sexual relationship with a 28-year-old man, but he has had no other partners in that time. He has insertive and receptive oral–genital, oral–anal, and peno-anal intercourse; condoms are used infrequently for anal intercourse and not at all for oral sex.

What Conditions May Cause His Symptoms?

The symptoms are strongly suggestive of acute hepatitis. The sexual transmission of hepatitis A and B viruses among men who have sex with men is well recognized, and infection with either virus must be considered in this case. Hepatitis C virus is also transmissible sexually but, with the exception of HIV-infected individuals, both the prevalence of infection among MSM and the risk of transmission are low. Less common causes of viral hepatitis include cytomegalovirus and Epstein–Barr virus infections. Hepatitis can also be a feature of secondary syphilis. Acute alcoholic hepatitis and drug-induced hepatitis can be excluded if the history is accurate. Rarer conditions such as Wilson's disease and autoimmune hepatitis need to be considered if viral hepatitis is excluded.

A. McMillan, *Sexually Transmissible Infections in Clinical Practice*,   203
DOI 10.1007/978-1-84882-557-4_32,
© Springer-Verlag London Limited 2009

TABLE 32.1. Results of laboratory tests.

Hematology:	Clinical biochemistry:
Hemoglobin: 146 g/L (130–180 g/L)[a]	Bilirubin: 46 μmol/L (2–17 μmol)
Mean corpuscular volume: 83 fL (78–98 fL)	Alanine aminotransferase (ALT): 900 U/L (10–50 U/L)
Leucocytes: 8.9×10^9/L (4.0–11.0 × 10^9/L)	Alkaline phosphatase: 180 U/L (40–125 U/L)
Differential white cell count:	Gamma glutamyl transferase: 92 U/L (5–55 U/L)
• *Neutrophil granulocytes:* 3.2×10^9/L (2.0–7.5 × 10^9/L)	
• *Lymphocytes:* 4.9×10^9/L (1.5–4.0 × 10^9/L)	Albumin: 36 g/L (35–50 g/L)
• *Monocytes:* 0.7×10^9/L (0.2–0.8 × 10^9/L)	
• Platelets: 148×10^9/L (150–350 × 10^9/L)	
• Prothrombin time: 13.5 s (8.0–10.5 s)	

[a]Reference values in parentheses.

Michael is not distressed. His sclerae and skin are yellow. His temperature is 37.1°C, and his pulse rate is 55 per minute. There is no significant superficial lymph node enlargement. The abdomen moves well with respiration. The liver is palpable 2 cm below the costal margin and is slightly tender; the spleen is not palpable. There are no other abnormal clinical findings. Table 32.1 shows the results of laboratory tests. How do you interpret these?

The results show a predominantly hepatocellular jaundice: the alanine aminotransferase is disproportionately elevated compared with the alkaline phosphatase and gamma glutamyl transferase (GGT). [1] A relative lymphocytosis is common in viral hepatitis, and the only mildly prolonged prothrombin time indicates mild liver damage.

Table 32.2 shows the results of the serological tests that his GP undertook. How do you interpret these?

---

[1]Disproportionately elevated alkaline phosphatase and GGT compared with alanine aminotransferase is seen when jaundice is caused by biliary obstruction.

TABLE 32.2. Results of serological tests for viral hepatitis, syphilis, and HIV.

Viral infection tested for:	Results
Hepatitis A	Anti-HAV IgM: NEGATIVE
	Anti-HAV IgG: POSITIVE
Hepatitis B	HBsAg: POSITIVE
	Anti-HBc IgG: POSITIVE
	Anti-HBc IgM: POSITIVE
	HBe antigen: POSITIVE
	Anti-HBe: NEGATIVE
	Anti-HBs: NEGATIVE
Hepatitis C	Anti-HCV: NEGATIVE
Cytomegalovirus	Anti-HCMV IgG: POSITIVE
	Anti-HCMV IgM: NEGATIVE
Epstein–Barr virus	Anti-EBV IgG: POSITIVE
	Anti-VCA IgM: NEGATIVE
Syphilis	Anti-treponemal EIA: NEGATIVE
HIV	Anti-HIV EIA: NEGATIVE

Key to abbreviations:
Anti-HAV: antibody against hepatitis A virus.
HBsAg: hepatitis B surface antigen.
Anti-HBc: antibody against hepatitis B core antigen.
Anti-HBs: antibody against hepatitis B surface antigen.
Anti-HCV: antibody against hepatitis C virus.
Anti-HCMV: antibody against human cytomegalovirus.
Anti-EBV: antibody against Epstein–Barr virus
Anti-VCA: antibody against Epstein–Barr virus capsid antigens.
EIA: Enzyme immunoassay.

There is clear evidence of acute hepatitis B infection: HBsAg is present in the plasma, and the IgM antibody response to hepatitis B core antigen is characteristic of acute infection. Although anti-HBc is found in chronic hepatitis B, it is of the IgG class, and not IgM. During the course of acute infection, antibody against hepatitis B surface antigen only becomes detectable during convalescence (Fig. 32.1).

The finding of IgG antibody against hepatitis A virus, cytomegalovirus, and Epstein–Barr virus indicates previous exposure to these agents; acute infection elicits an IgM response.

The negative screening test (anti-treponemal EIA) excludes a diagnosis of secondary syphilis.

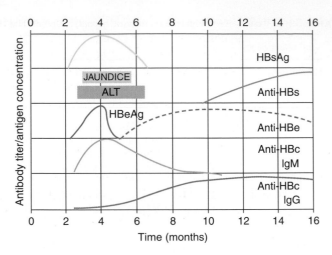

FIGURE 32.1. Serological events observed during acute hepatitis B virus infection.

How Is Hepatitis B Transmitted?

Hepatitis B virus (HBV) is transmitted parenterally, and, for example, may be transmitted as a result of inoculation of minute quantities of blood as may occur during intravenous drug use, if care is not taken to sterilize the needles or other equipment. For some time it has been known that MSM are at risk of HBV infection. Practices likely to result in mucosal trauma, including genital–anal and oral–anal intercourse and rectal douching, correlate with the presence of HBV serological markers. Vaccination should therefore be offered to all sexually active MSM who are not known to be immune to the infection (serum anti-HBs negative) (see Case 3).

What Clinical Features May Be Associated with Acute Hepatitis B Virus Infection?

Many cases of hepatitis B are symptomless and detectable only by biochemical tests for hepatocellular damage. In those who develop clinical manifestations of the disease, following an incubation period of 40–160 days, there is a pre-icteric stage (prodrome) during which the symptoms of the disease develop. The patient complains of nausea, malaise, anorexia, and discomfort in the upper right abdomen. Tender enlargement of the liver is found in most cases, and in about 20% of patients the spleen is also enlarged. Other, less common clinical features include erythematous, maculopapular or urticarial skin rash, and arthralgia.

Although Not the Causes of the Hepatitis in this Case, How are Hepatitis A, Cytomegalovirus and Epstein–Barr Virus Transmitted?

Hepatitis A virus (HAV) is transmitted by the fecal–oral route. The virus is excreted in the feces and infection is usually acquired orally under conditions of poor hygiene and sanitation. Most studies have shown that the prevalence of antibody against HAV is significantly higher in the sera of homosexual men than in heterosexual men who attend STD clinics. The occurrence of outbreaks of hepatitis A among MSM also supports the conclusion that such men are at increased risk of infection. The acquisition of hepatitis A correlates with a large number of sexual partners and frequent oral–anal sexual contact. Vaccination is therefore routinely offered to sexually active MSM who have no serological evidence of prior infection (serum anti-HAV IgG negative).

The majority of infections with HAV are symptomless. When symptomatic, the clinical and biochemical features of hepatitis A are similar to those of any other viral hepatitis (see above). The incubation period of hepatitis A varies between 30 and 50 days. In general the course of the illness is shorter and less severe than that of hepatitis B, with resolution of both clinical and biochemical abnormalities within 1 month of onset of the illness.

Human cytomegalovirus (HCMV) is usually acquired in early childhood probably from contact with infected secretions from infected children. Mother-to-child transmission is important as congenital infection can lead to considerable morbidity. The virus is found in semen, and there is good evidence for sexual transmission of. The prevalence of HCMV antibodies is higher among

MSM than among men who have sex with women. Transmission via blood or blood products or transplanted tissues is also possible.

Although most infections with EBV are acquired through kissing, the virus can be transmitted sexually, possibly by oral–genital contact, but perhaps also from the male genital tract. There is no evidence that EBV infection is more prevalent among MSM than the general population.

What Is the Course of Acute Hepatitis B, and How Would You Manage This Man?

With the development of jaundice, the patient's condition improves and within 2–4 weeks most infections have resolved. Uncommonly (<1% of cases), acute liver failure develops within 4 weeks of the onset of symptoms. The mortality rate of acute hepatitis B is less than 1%. Individuals who have symptomatic acute hepatitis B are likely to clear the virus, the risk of developing chronic hepatitis being <10%; this risk, however, is increased if the person is HIV infected.

In most cases, acute hepatitis B virus infection is a self-limiting condition, and there is no specific therapy. The development of hepatic decompensation (somnolence or change of personality) necessitates admission to hospital and referral to a hepatologist for specialist management. Other than the avoidance of alcohol during the acute illness and convalescence, dietary restrictions are unnecessary. He should be advised about the risks of sexual transmission, and he should avoid unprotected sexual intercourse, oral–anal, and oral–genital contact until he has become HBsAg negative and anti-HBs positive, or his sexual partner(s) have been successfully vaccinated (anti-HBs >100 mIU/L).

Michael should be offered screening for other sexually transmitted infections (see Case 4).

He should be reviewed at 2-weekly intervals until the alanine (and aspartate) aminotransferase level is normal.

His parents and sister should be offered an accelerated course of recombinant hepatitis B vaccine (see Case 3), and Michael's partner should be asked to attend for screening, and, if indicated, vaccination.

TABLE 32.3. Results of serological tests for hepatitis B in the patient's sexual partner.

HBsAg: POSITIVE
Anti-HBc IgG: POSITIVE
Anti-HBc IgM: NEGATIVE
HBeAg: POSITIVE
Anti-HBe: NEGATIVE
Anti-HBs: NEGATIVE

Michael's partner, Sam, attends a sexual health clinic the day after Michael is told the diagnosis. He is symptomless, and he has never felt the need to attend such a clinic before because, until he met Michael, anal intercourse had always been protected. He has not been vaccinated against hepatitis B. Clinical examination is unremarkable; in particular there are no signs of chronic liver disease. Table 32.3 shows the results of serological testing for hepatitis B. His ALT is 72 U/L. An HIV antibody/antigen test is negative.

How Do You Interpret These Results?

The pattern of serological tests and the mildly elevated ALT suggest that he is a chronic carrier of HBV (immune active). As such patients are at high risk of disease progression with the development of cirrhosis and hepatocellular carcinoma, referral to a hepatologist is recommended.

Case 33
A Pregnant Woman Who is a Contact of a Man with Infectious Syphilis

Charles's wife (Case 19), who is 4 month's pregnant joins her hus-band in the United Kingdom 1 week after he is diagnosed as having secondary syphilis. He tells her his diagnosis and persuades her to attend the Sexual Health clinic.

What Are the Risks of Untreated Early Syphilis in a Pregnant Woman?

Infection of the fetus is more likely to occur when the mother's infection is in the early stage, as at this time considerable numbers of treponemes are present in the circulation. During the first year of infection in an untreated woman there is an 80–90% probability that the infection will be transmitted to the fetus. The chance of fetal infection declines rapidly after the second year of infection in the mother and becomes rare after the fourth year. In general, the greater the duration of syphilis in the mother, the less chance there is of the fetus being affected. If a mother with early-stage syphilis is not treated, 25–30% of fetuses die in utero; 25–30% die after birth; and of the infected survivors 40% develop late symptomatic syphilis.

Charles's wife attends the clinic. She is symptomless, and in par-ticular she has not noticed any genital lesions suggestive of infec-tion. The pregnancy is progressing satisfactorily. There is no past history of syphilis. She has documented allergy to penicillin. Clin-ical examination confirms the absence of external genital ulcer-ation, and lesions of the vagina or uterine cervix are not found.

A. McMillan, *Sexually Transmissible Infections in Clinical Practice*, 211
DOI 10.1007/978-1-84882-557-4_33,
© Springer-Verlag London Limited 2009

TABLE 33.1. Results of serological tests for syphilis at initial clinic attendance.

Screening anti-treponemal EIA[a]: POSITIVE
Venereal Diseases Research Laboratory (VDRL) test: POSITIVE at a titer of 4
Treponema pallidum particle agglutination test (TPPA): POSITIVE at a titer of 2560
Anti-treponemal IgM EIA[a]: POSITIVE

[a]Enzyme immunoassay.

Serological tests for treponemal infection are performed and the results are shown in Table 33.1.

An HIV antigen/antibody EIA is negative.

How Do You Interpret These Results?

These results confirm treponemal infection, and as she is a recent sexual contact of a man with secondary syphilis, the diagnosis of early-latent infection is made.

Note: The endemic treponematoses – yaws, pinta, and endemic syphilis (bejel) – that are transmissible by direct skin contact most commonly infect young children produce results in the serological tests from syphilis that resemble those found in venereal syphilis. Yaws, caused by *Treponema pallidum,* subspecies *pertenue*, is found in tropical Africa. Endemic syphilis, caused by *Treponema pallidum* subspecies *endemicum*, occurs in the Arabian peninsula and along the southern border of the Sahara desert, and pinta, caused by *Treponema carateum* is found in scattered foci in northern South America. It may not be possible to differentiate the non-venereal treponematoses from venereal syphilis in individuals from geographical areas where these infections are prevalent, and in whom there are no clinical features of past or current infection. It is better to treat the person as if he or she had syphilis.

How Would You Treat This Patient?

Treatment of pregnant women with syphilis who are allergic to penicillin is difficult. The tetracyclines are contraindicated in

TABLE 33.2. Results of serological tests for syphilis before delivery.

Screening anti-treponemal enzyme immunoassay (EIA): POSITIVE
Venereal Disease Research Laboratory (VDRL) test: NEGATIVE
Treponema pallidum particle agglutination (TPPA) test: POSITIVE at
   a titer of 640
Anti-treponemal IgM EIA: NEGATIVE

pregnancy. Ceftriaxone has been used in the treatment of small numbers of patients with early syphilis with apparent success. However, there are concerns about cross-hypersensitivity with the penicillins (see Case 28). Treatment failures have been described following treatment with erythromycin. Although azithromycin has been used in the treatment of pregnant women with syphilis, efficacy is uncertain, and infection with strains of *Treponema pallidum* that are resistant to the macrolides is well documented. It is recommended that babies born to mothers who have been treated with the macrolides should be treated with penicillin after birth. For this reason, desensitization to penicillin is recommended followed by treatment with penicillin.

Charles's wife is admitted to hospital for desensitizing to penicillin and is treated with benzathine penicillin thereafter. She is followed-up at monthly intervals with clinical examination and serological testing. Two weeks before delivery, the results of serological tests are shown in Table 33.2 .

How Do You Interpret These Results, and How Would You Manage the Neonate?

These results are in keeping with adequately treated early syphilis (see Case 19). (A four-fold rise in VDRL titer would have been an indication for re-treatment). However, follow-up of the newborn child is recommended with clinical examination and the undertaking of serological tests to ensure that the child is uninfected.

The diagnosis of congenital syphilis can be difficult because most affected neonates are symptomless at birth. The screening EIA, the VDRL test, and the TPPA may be positive in the neonate's blood in the absence of active infection. The IgG found in the serum of neonates is largely passively acquired through the placenta and does not represent the infant's own response. A rising or higher titer in the neonate's blood than in the mother is suggestive of infection; lower titers in neonates when compared to their mothers are suggestive of passively transferred antibody. In the absence of infection passively transferred antibody detected by the VDRL (or rapid plasma regain test [RPR]) will decrease and the tests will become negative in approximately 3 months. In the case of the treponemal antigen tests it may take up to 6 or 9 months for the test to become negative. The demonstration of anti-treponemal IgM in neonatal serum correlates well with congenital infection. Because of the possibility of a delayed IgM response or suppression of IgM synthesis in the neonate due to high levels of circulating maternal anti-treponemal IgG, IgM testing should be repeated after 4, 8, and 12 weeks.

Case 34
An HIV-Infected Man with Anal Pain, Anal Discharge, and Bleeding

A 32-year-old man, Frank, presents to a Sexual Health clinic with a 1-week history of pain in the perianal region, a discharge of thick yellow material from the anal canal, a feeling of incomplete bowel emptying, and bleeding after defecation. There are no other symptoms, in particular he has not noticed fever and there has been no abdominal pain. He is HIV infected, the diagnosis having been made 5 years previously. He has never been treated with antiretroviral drugs, and he gives no history of illicit use of such agents. A baseline genotypic assay did not identify mutations in the HIV genome likely to confer resistance to antiviral drugs. His CD4+ T-cell count was 467 per mm^3 (normal range 500–1500 per mm^3) and a plasma viral HIV concentration of 7,853 copies per mL when he was tested about 12 weeks previously. Over the past 7 years he has had six episodes of rectal and urethral gonorrhoea, three episodes of rectal chlamydial infection (the infecting genotype was unknown), and numerous infections with pubic lice. Two years previously he was treated for primary syphilis of the anal canal with two injections of benzathine penicillin, given at a week's interval. One year after treatment, the Venereal Diseases Research Laboratory (VDRL) test was negative, an anti-treponemal IgM enzyme immunoassay was negative, and the Treponema pallidum *particle agglutination (TPPA) test was weakly positive, with a titer of 40, this pattern of results being consistent with adequately treated early syphilis.*

When he attended for a sexual health screen about 5 years previously, it was noted that he had had prior infection with hepatitis B virus: hepatitis B surface antigen was negative, but anti-core

A. McMillan, *Sexually Transmissible Infections in Clinical Practice*, 215
DOI 10.1007/978-1-84882-557-4_34,
© Springer-Verlag London Limited 2009

antibody was detected. As there was no serological evidence of prior exposure to hepatitis A, he completed a course of hepatitis A vaccine at that time. He has no past history of gastrointestinal disease.

He has a regular partner with whom he has had an open relationship for more than 3 years. His partner is also HIV-infected and is not receiving antiviral therapy. They have unprotected receptive and insertive anal intercourse with each other and with most of their numerous casual sexual contacts. The most recent occasion on which they had sex was at a party in Berlin, Germany, about 6 weeks previously. Both had unprotected receptive anal sex with five different men, and Frank also participated in insertive and receptive "fisting"[1] with one man. He regularly uses oral amphetamines and inhales nitrites during anal sex, but he has never injected drugs.

What Diagnoses Do You Consider?

The symptoms are consistent with those of a distal proctitis. Table 20.1 (Case 20) indicates the causes of a distal proctitis. In the case presented here, infection with *Chlamydia trachomatis* genotypes D–K is an unlikely cause of such severe symptoms: most infected individuals, if symptomatic, have mild features of distal proctitis. Lymphogranuloma venereum (LGV) genotypes, however, can cause severe proctitis, and, as there have been recent outbreaks of such infection in Western Europe, this is the most likely diagnosis. Gonococcal proctitis can be severe as can primary herpetic infection, particularly in the immunocompromised. Syphilis, of course, needs to be considered. Peri-rectal cellulitis can result from receptive "fisting," extra-peritoneal rupture of the rectum allowing passage of bacteria into the tissues surrounding the rectum. However, most cases present within a few days of the risk, and abdominal pain and fever are usual.

He looks well but is in considerable discomfort. His temperature is 37.2°C, and his pulse is 75 per minute. Other than mild seborrhoeic dermatitis of the chest wall, there are no abnormal

---

[1]"Fisting" (synonyms: fist fornication, brachioproctic eroticism) is the insertion of a closed hand through the anal canal into the distal rectum.

dermatological findings. His abdomen moves well with respiration, and there is no tenderness or guarding; neither the liver nor the spleen is palpable. There is significant enlargement (>1 cm in diameter) of the posterior cervical, axillary, and inguinal lymph nodes that are not tender. The external genitalia and the perianal region appear normal. During anoscopy, a copious mucopurulent discharge is found within the distal rectum. The rectal mucosa is edematous with loss of the normal vascular pattern. The mucosa bleeds easily, and several small ulcers, about 5 mm in diameter are noted. These inflammatory changes, however, do not extend beyond the rectosigmoid junction.

How Do the Clinical Findings Aid the Differential Diagnosis?

Generalized lymph node enlargement is a feature of HIV infection, and its finding here may reflect this and not superadded infection such as syphilis. Seborrhoeic dermatitis is common among HIV-infected individuals. The absence of perianal ulceration argues against, but does not exclude, a diagnosis of primary anorectal herpes. The anoscopy findings confirm proctitis. The sexually transmitted organisms shown in Table 20.1 (Case 20) cause proctitis that is generally confined to the distal 12–15 cm of the rectum. Inflammatory changes extending more proximally would alert the physician to a diagnosis of proctocolitis, as may occur in infection with *Shigella* spp., *Campylobacter* spp, and *Entamoeba histolytica*, the causative organism of amoebic dysentery.[2]

Specimens are taken for the diagnosis or exclusion of gonococcal and chlamydial infections as described in Case 4. A Gram-stained smear of rectal material shows many polymorphonuclear leucocytes, but Gram-negative diplococci are not identified. As LGV proctitis is a possible diagnosis, the microbiology laboratory is alerted to this possibility and if chlamydiae are identified by a

---

[2]Infection with the non-pathogenic protozoan *Entamoeba dispar* that resembles *Entamoeba histolytica* microscopically is common among men who have sex with men. It is therefore important to differentiate the species before making an erroneous diagnosis of amoebiasis in a man with intestinal symptoms.

nucleic acid amplification assay, genotyping is requested. Mate-rial from the rectal ulcers is obtained using a cotton wool-tipped applicator stick and sent in viral transport medium for the detec-tion of herpes simplex virus DNA (see Case 16). A further sample from the ulcers is sent for testing for T. pallidum *DNA by a poly-merase chain reaction. In addition, serological tests for syphilis are undertaken, and as 3 months had elapsed since his most recent HIV evaluation, blood is obtained for routine hematological and biochemical tests, the CD4⁺ T-cell count, HIV plasma viral load, and screening for hepatitis C virus infection.*

What Is Your Immediate Management of This Case?

In this case, the symptoms are of a severity that empirical treatment is indicated (Table 34.1).

Although Gram-negative diplococci are not seen in the smear, this test has a sensitivity of only between 70 and 80%, and the regimen used should therefore include an agent to treat gonococcal infection.

As herpetic proctitis cannot be excluded on clinical grounds, it is justified to include valaciclovir in the drug regimen.

Frank is treated with ceftriaxone, doxycycline, and valaciclovir, and he re-attends the clinic 1 week later. His symptoms have improved considerably. The results of the laboratory tests are now available (Table 34.2).

How Do You Interpret These Results?

The detection of a *C. trachomatis* LGV genotype strongly supports the diagnosis of LGV proctitis. Although most infected individu-als have symptoms and signs of a severe proctitis, some patients, probably a minority, with LGV rectal infection are symptomless and finding in this case may be co-incidental.

TABLE 34.1. Antimicrobial drug regimens for the empirical treatment of moderate-to-severe distal proctitis caused by sexually transmitted infections (The 2007 European Guideline [International Union Against Sexually Transmitted Infections/World Health Organization] on the management of proctitis, proctocolitis, and enteritis caused by sexually transmitted pathogens).

Ceftriaxone 250 mg as a single intramuscular injection
OR
Cefotaxime 100 mg as a single intramuscular injection
OR
Cefixime 400 mg as a single oral dose
OR
Cefuroxime axetil 1000 mg as a single oral dose[a]
PLUS
Doxycycline 100 mg twice daily by mouth for 21 days
OR
Tetracycline 500 mg four times per day by mouth for 21 days
OR
Erythromycin base 500 mg four times per day by mouth for 21 days
PLUS
Valaciclovir 500 mg twice daily by mouth for 5–10 days

[a]Second-line oral therapy.

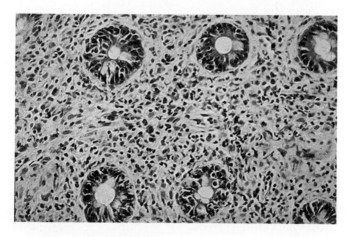

FIGURE 34.1. Granulomatous proctitis caused by lymphogranuloma venereum, genotype L-2.

The genotypes of LGV attack lymphatic and sub-epithelial tissues rather that the epithelial cells as occurs with infection with the oculogenital genotypes of *C. trachomatis*. The former invade the epithelial cells within which multiplication occurs with the release of elementary bodies from the basal cell surface to invade the underlying tissues. As a result, there is destruction of the mucosa and transmural inflammation of the rectal wall. There is also involvement of the regional lymph nodes. The histology as

TABLE 34.2. Results of laboratory tests.

Investigations	Result
Microbiology	
NAAT[a] for *Chlamydia trachomatis*	POSITIVE: genotype L2a
NAAT[a] for *Neisseria gonorrhoeae*	NEGATIVE
PCR[b] for herpes simplex virus	NEGATIVE
PCR[b] for *Treponema pallidum*	NEGATIVE
Serological tests for syphilis	VDRL[c]: POSITIVE, titer 512
	TPPA[d]: POSITIVE, titer >5120
	Anti-treponemal IgM: POSITIVE
Anti-HCV[e]	NEGATIVE
Biochemical tests on serum	
Bilirubin	9 μmol/L (normal <17 μmol/L)
Alanine aminotransferase (ALT)	708 Units/L (normal range 5–30 Units/L)
Alkaline phosphatase	161 Units/L (normal range 25–110 Units/L)
CD4$^+$ T-cell count	243 per mm^3
Plasma HIV viral load	86,000 per mL

[a]Nucleic acid amplification test.
[b]Polymerase chain reaction.
[c]Venereal Diseases Research Laboratory test.
[d]*Treponema pallidum* particle agglutination assay.
[e]Hepatitis C virus.

noted in rectal biopsies (Fig. 34.1) is similar to that found in Crohn's disease: infiltration of the lamina propria with lymphocytes, plasma cells, and histiocytes with crypt abscess and granuloma formation. Indeed many cases in the recent western European outbreak of LGV proctitis were initially treated for inflammatory bowel disease for several months before the true diagnosis was made.

The serological findings indicate that Frank has become re-infected with syphilis: (a) there is seroconversion from a negative VDRL test to one with a high titer, (b) the TPPA shows a significant increase in titer (more than eight-fold), and (c) the anti-treponemal IgM test is positive. (The non-treponemal tests for syphilis VDRL or the rapid plasma regain [RPR] are the most sensitive for detecting re-infection with *T. pallidum*). In some HIV-infected individuals high VDRL or RPR titers are found. Although the anti-treponemal IgM EIA was positive in this man, in at least one-third of re-infections this test is negative.

Syphilis can cause a distal proctitis, and, despite a negative PCR for *T. pallidum*, it cannot be entirely excluded as contributing to the disease process in this case.

The plasma enzyme tests of liver function are abnormal with a hepatitic pattern – the ALT is raised disproportionately compared with the alkaline phosphatase. Among HIV-infected individuals, abnormal liver function tests may be caused by a variety of opportunistic infections, including cytomegalovirus and *Cryptosporidium* spp. In this case, however, the patient is only mildly immuno-compromised, and such opportunistic infections would be unusual. As he had been vaccinated previously against hepatitis A, this is an unlikely cause of hepatitis in this case. However, an anti-hepatitis A IgM test should be requested. Re-activation of hepatitis B infection has been documented in HIV-infected individuals, and repeat serological testing and a specific HBV DNA NAAT should be requested. Although the antibody test for hepatitis C virus is negative, early infection with that virus cannot be excluded as a cause of his abnormal liver function tests. A polymerase chain reaction assay should be requested to detect HCV RNA as it is detectable in the plasma several weeks before an antibody response is observed. Early syphilis, particularly secondary disease, can be associated with hepatitis. In most case reports, however, the alkaline phosphatase is disproportionately elevated compared with the transaminases. Non-Hodgkin's lymphoma and Kaposi's sarcoma can also affect the liver, and such conditions need to be considered in the differential diagnosis.

There are several explanations for the decline in the CD4$^+$ T-cell count in the peripheral blood, and the increased viral load compared 3 months previously. A change in the assay systems used may account for these changes. Alternatively, intercurrent infection, for example, with syphilis, can result in these changes. A particular concern is that he has become infected with another strain of HIV. As he has had unprotected receptive and insertive anal intercourse with multiple partners, this is a plausible explanation. It is known that individuals who become super-infected with HIV progress more rapidly to a severely immunocompromised state. There is also the possibility of infection with drug-resistant virus, making the choice of future antiretroviral therapy more difficult.

Hepatitis C virus RNA is detected in a plasma sample. A genotypic resistance assay performed on his plasma HIV shows mutations likely to confer resistance to the non-nucleoside reverse transcriptase inhibitors nevirapine and efavirenz.

Hepatitis C virus is usually acquired by the parenteral route, particularly among infecting drug users. The risk of sexual transmission has generally been considered to be low, with the possible exception of HIV-infected individuals in whom the concentration of HCV in plasma and genital secretions may be high. However, outbreaks of acute hepatitis C have been described among men who have sex with men in whom other risk factors, such as injecting drug use, have not been identified. Many of these men have had multiple sexual partners, have had unprotected receptive and insertive anal intercourse, have participated in "fisting," have been treated previously for STIs, and have participated in group sex. This patient matches such a profile. Mucosal damage from "fisting" and LGV has been shown to facilitate transmission of this virus.

The absence of resistance mutations in the baseline sample and lack of a history of taking antiretroviral medication, either prescribed or illicitly, suggests that he has subsequently acquired resistant virus. In some circles, antiretroviral drugs are shared in the mistaken notion that they will prevent acquisition of HIV during unprotected sexual contact. This does not appear to be the case here.

Frank continues on treatment with doxycycline for 21 days. Although doxycycline is a treatment for syphilis, cure is less certain than with penicillin, and he is therefore treated with benzathine penicillin (see Case 11).[3] He is referred to a hepatologist for management of his acute hepatitis C. Follow-up to ensure cure of the LGV and syphilis is arranged. In addition, further one-to-one counseling about his high-risk behavior is undertaken.

---

[3] Some physicians treat early syphilis in an HIV-infected patient as if he/she had neuosyphilis: procaine penicillin G 2 g by intramuscular injection daily for 17 days PLUS probenecid 500 mg four times per day by mouth for 17 days.

Case 35
A Young Girl with Anogenital Lumps

Claire is a 15-month-old girl who has been brought by her mother to you as her General Practitioner. While bathing Claire, the mother had noted lumps in the anogenital area. When you examine her, you note the presence of anogenital warts (Fig. 35.1).

How Do You Explain the Presence of Anogenital Warts in a Pre-pubertal Child, and What History Would You Wish to Elicit from the Mother?

The presence of anogenital warts in a pre-pubertal child can be explained in several ways. These include

- perinatal acquisition of anogenital warts from a clinically or sub-clinically infected mother;
- inoculation with a common wart virus type on the child's genitals by auto-inoculation or during routine handling by a carer; and
- infection transmitted during child sexual abuse (CSA).

The most common explanation is perinatal transmission of anogenital warts from mother to child (this includes transplacental transmission). Anogenital warts thus acquired commonly manifest in the first year of life, though their appearance may be delayed for up to 2–3 years after birth. These mothers often, though not invariably, have a past history of anogenital warts. It is possible for wart virus types causing hand warts (e.g., HPV types 1, 2, and 4, etc.) to be transmitted to a child's genitals by auto-inoculation or by carers during routine care, though this is very uncommon. The various HPV types causing warts are generally anatomical site specific,

A. McMillan, *Sexually Transmissible Infections in Clinical Practice*,
DOI 10.1007/978-1-84882-557-4_35,
© Springer-Verlag London Limited 2009

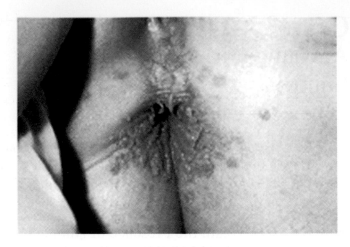

FIGURE 35.1. Anogenital warts in a young girl.

and it is unusual for non-genital wart virus types to infect anogenital skin. Finally, the possibility of child sexual abuse as a potential explanation for anogenital warts in a minor must also always be kept in mind.

The mother should be carefully questioned regarding any personal history of previous genital warts, and especially any history of genital warts during pregnancy. If the child's genital warts appear to be similar to common skin warts, enquiries should be made as to whether the child herself, the mother, or other carers currently have hand warts. If sexual abuse is considered a possibility, details of all adults with responsibility for the child's care should be ascertained.

Where a pre-pubertal child has genital warts, because of the requirement to consider possibility of sexual abuse, General Practitioners faced with this scenario should request specialist involvement.

What Investigations Might You Consider in This Case, and with Which Agencies Might You Wish to Liase?

Child protection issues arise when a diagnosis of a sexually transmissible infection in a pre-pubertal child is made. A multi-agency approach must be adopted from the outset, and the social work department and community pediatricians involved, as well as consulting Sexual Health physicians. Following discussion with these agencies, it may also be necessary to involve the police.

Where the possibility of sexual abuse has been raised, a careful forensic physical and genital examination of the child must be carried out, looking specifically for signs of abuse. The timing of the forensic examination is important and is dependent upon the time period the alleged abuse. Testing must also be performed for all relevant sexually transmitted infections, using a "chain of evidence" protocol, by a clinician experienced in this field. The timing of the STI screen is also important and is dependent upon the pre-patent period of the STIs, as well as the time period of the alleged abuse. Where appropriate (for example, where the alleged abuse has occurred over a lengthy period) the forensic examination and STI screen can be performed together on a single occasion.

The STI screen in pre-pubertal girls usually includes testing for *Chlamydia trachomatis, Neisseria gonorrhoeae*, and *Trichomonas vaginalis*. Where there is definitive evidence or disclosure regarding sexual abuse, consideration must be given to sampling all possible sites of abuse for relevant infections. Where there is only a suspicion of abuse, sampling sites need to be decided on a case-by-case basis, depending on history, symptoms, signs, and the probability of abuse having been perpetrated.

Chlamydia trachomatis can infect the vagina of pre-pubertal girls, as well as the oro-pharynx and rectum, and these sites need to be sampled depending on the abuse history (as discussed above). Urethral sampling is usually avoided due to poor tolerance of minors for this test. In these circumstances, testing a first-voided urine sample should be considered. A sample of vaginal discharge, if present, should be obtained or specimens collected from the posterior wall of the vagina or from the introitus. Care must be taken to avoid the hymen, if present, to prevent unnecessary discomfort to the child. Trans-hymenal swabs can be taken if the size of the hymenal opening allows this. The swabs used for sampling ear, nose, and throat sites should be used for trans-hymenal sampling as they are smaller than the cotton tipped swabs routinely used for STI screening.

Although nucleic acid amplification tests (NAAT) for *Chlamydia trachomatis* are unlicensed for use on specimens obtained from children, they are now commonly used because of their high sensitivity in adults. A positive NAAT in a child must be confirmed either by culture (preferably, but culture facilities are rarely available in many laboratories) or by a different NAAT to increase result validity for medico-legal purposes. Interpretation of NAAT testing should be done in collaboration with genitourinary medicine specialists and microbiologists, taking into account the anatomical site sampled and local prevalence data which affect the test's positive and negative predictive values.

Neisseria gonorrhoeae can also infect the vagina, oropharynx, and rectum of pre-pubertal girls and consideration should be given to sampling these sites depending on the history of abuse. Culture remains the gold standard laboratory investigation for *N. gonorrhoeae* for medico-legal purposes. Nucleic acid amplification tests for *N. gonorrhoeae* can be undertaken in addition or if urine testing if being performed, but a positive NAAT result will require confirmation by culture.

Vaginal swabs should be taken for microscopy and, if facilities are available, for culture or use of a NAAT for *Trichomonas vaginalis*. If any vaginal discharge is present, consider microscopy and culture for *Candida* spp. and bacterial vaginosis. If there is genital ulceration, samples for testing for herpes simplex virus infection by polymerase chain reaction or culture should be obtained.

Serological testing for syphilis, HIV, Hepatitis B, and Hepatitis C should be undertaken, depending on the risk factors. The samples may require to be repeated if initial testing is undertaken within the window period of the infections. Very rarely, depending on the period, timing and type of sexual abuse, and the risk of blood-borne virus infections, vaccination for Hepatitis B and post-exposure prophylaxis for HIV may be appropriate.

How Would You Treat These Warts?

As anogenital warts will spontaneously regress, treatment should only be considered after a lapse of at least 3 months. When the warts are causing significant symptoms (e.g., bleeding or bacterial superinfection), treatment may need to be initiated earlier.

Antimitotic treatments such as podophyllotoxin and 5-fluorouracil and immune-modulators (imiquimod) are not licensed in children. Occasionally, under specialist guidance, podophyllotoxin can be used in children over the age of 2 years. Anogenital warts in a minor can be treated with cryotherapy, scissor excision, or electrosurgery. These treatments are often very poorly tolerated in young children and may need to be carried out under general anesthesia.

Further Reading

General

Adler MW, Cowan F, French P, Mitchell H, Richens J. *ABC of Sexually Transmitted Infections*. 2004. London. BMJ Publications. 104 pp.

Clutterbuck D. *Specialist Training in Sexually Transmitted Infections and HIV*. 2004. Amsterdam. Elsevier. 304 pp.

Holmes KK, Sparling PF, Stamm WE, Piot P, Wasserheit JN, Corey L, Cohen MS, Watts DH (eds). *Sexually Transmitted Diseases*. 4th edn. 2008. New York. McGraw-Hill Companies Ltd. 2166 pp.

Guidelines

Centers for Disease control and Prevention. Sexually Transmitted Diseases Guidelines, 2006. *MMWR* 2006; **55** (No. RR 11): 33–35.

BASHH Clinical Effectiveness Group Guidelines. www.bashh.org/guidelines

Case 5

Ross JDC, Jensen JS. *Mycoplasma genitalium* as a sexually transmitted infection: implications for screening, testing, and treatment. *Sex Transm Infect* 2006; **82**: 269–271.

Bradshaw CS, Jensen JS, Tabrizi SN, et al. Azithromycin failure in *Mycoplasma genitalium* urethritis. *Emerg Infect Dis* 2006; **12**: 1149–1152.

A. McMillan, *Sexually Transmissible Infections in Clinical Practice*, 231
DOI 10.1007/978-1-84882-557-4_BM2,
© Springer-Verlag London Limited 2009

Case 11

Sobel JD. Vulvovaginal candidosis. *Lancet* 2007; **369**: 1961–1971.

Case 14

Low N, Egger M, Sterne JAC, et al. Incidence of severe reproductive tract complications associated with diagnosed genital chlamydial infection: the Uppsala Women's Cohort Study. *Sex Transm Infect* 2006; **82**: 212–218.

Case 15

Goon P, Sonnex C. Frequently asked questions about genital warts in the genitourinary medicine clinic: an update and review of recent literature. *Sex Transm Infect* 2008; **84**: 3–7.

Cutts FT, Franceschi S, Goldie S, et al. Human papillomavirus and HPV vaccines: a review. *Bull WHO* 2007; **85**: 719–726.

Case 16

Gupta R, Warren T, Wald A. Genital herpes. *Lancet* 2008; **370**: 2127–2137.

Case 20

McMillan A, van Voorst Vader PC, de Vries HJ. The 2007 European Guideline (International Union Against Sexually Transmitted Infections/World Health Organization) on the management of proctitis, proctocolitis and enteritis caused by sexually transmitted pathogens. *Int J STD AIDS* 2007; **18**: 514–520.

Case 21

Zetola NM, Pilcher CD. Diagnosis and management of acute HIV infection. *Infect Dis Clin N Amer* 2007; **21**: 19–48.

Case 22

Bradshaw CS, Tabrizi SN, Read TRH, et al. Etiologies of nongonococcal urethritis: bacteria, viruses, and the association with orogenital exposure. *J Infect Dis* 2006; **193**: 336–345.

Case 23

Braun J, Sieper J. Spondyloarthritides and related arthritides. In: Warrell DA, Cox TM, Firth JD, Benz EJ, eds. *Oxford Textbook of Medicine.* 4th edn. 2003. Oxford. Oxford University press. 3.43–3.53.

Gaston JSH. Reactive arthritis. In: Warrell DA, Cox TM, Firth JD, Benz EJ, eds. *Oxford Textbook of Medicine*. 4th edn. 2003. Oxford: Oxford University press. 3.57–3.61.

Shirliff ME, Mader JT. Acute septic arthritis. *Clin Microbiol Rev* 2002; **15**: 527–544.

Cases 24 and 25

See Case 11.

Case 27

Blas MM, Canchihuaman FA, Alva IE, Hawes SE. Pregnancy outcomes in women infected with *Chlamydia trachomatis*: a population-based cohort study in Washington State. *Sex Transm Infect* 2007; **83**: 314–318.

Morse SA, Beck-Sague CM. Gonorrhoea. In: Hitchcock PJ, MacKay HT, Wasserheit JN, eds. *Sexually Transmitted Diseases and Adverse Outcomes of Pregnancy*. 1999. Washington DC. ASM Press. 151–174.

Pitsouni E, Iavazzo C, Athanasiou S, Falagas ME. Single-dose azithromycin versus erythromycin or amoxicillin for *Chlamydia trachomatis* infection during pregnancy: a meta-analysis of randomised controlled trials. *Int J Antimicrob Agents* 2007; **30**: 213–221.

Case 28

National Guideline for the Management of Genital Herpes. 2007. Clinical Effectiveness Group (British Association for Sexual Health and HIV). www.bashh.org/guidelines/2002/hsv_ 0601.pdf

Hollier LM, Wendel GD. Third trimester antiviral prophylaxis for preventing maternal genital herpes simplex virus (HSV) recurrences and neonatal infection. The Cochrane Database of Systematic Reviews. 2008.

Case 29

Silverberg MJ, Thorsen P, Lindeberg H, Grant LA, Shah KV. Condyloma in pregnancy is strongly predictive of juvenile-onset recurrent respiratory papillomatosis. *Obstet Gynecol* 2003; **101**: 645–652.

Case 32

Centers for Disease control and Prevention. Sexually Transmitted Diseases Guidelines, 2006. *MMWR* 2006; **55** (No. RR 11): 33–35.

Case 33

Gotz HM, van Doornum G, Niesters HGM, den Hollander JG, Thio HB, de Zwart O. A cluster of acute hepatitis C virus infection among men who have sex with men – results from contact tracing and public health implications. *AIDS* 2005; **19**: 969–974.

McMillan A, van Voorst Vader PC, de Vries HJ. The 2007 European Guideline (International Union Against Sexually Transmitted Infections/World Health Organization) on the management of proctitis, proctocolitis and enteritis caused by sexually transmitted pathogens. *Int J STD AIDS* 2007; **18**: 514–520.

Nieuwenhuis RF, Ossewaarde JM, Gotz HM, et al. Resurgence of lymphogranuloma venereum in Western Europe: an outbreak of *Chlamydia trachomatis* serovar L2 proctitis in The Netherlands among men who have sex with men. *Clin Inf Dis* 2004; **39**: 996–1003.

Index

Note: The page numbers followed with the letter 't' and 'f' in the index denote the tables and figures.